James Duigan's
Blueprint
for Health

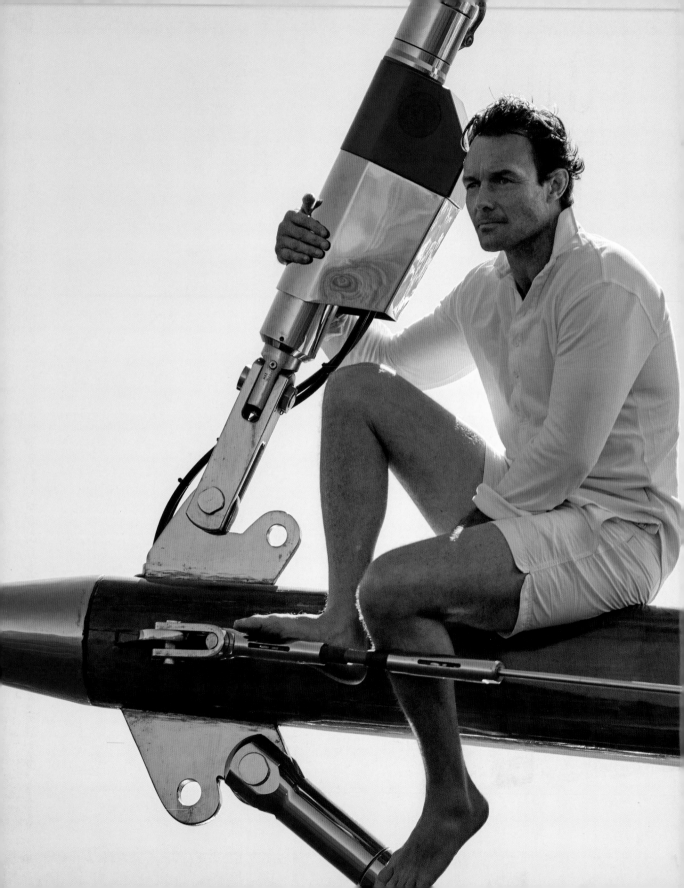

James Duigan's
Blueprint
for Health

LOSE WEIGHT
AND FEEL
BETTER IN
14 DAYS

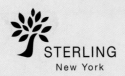

STERLING
New York

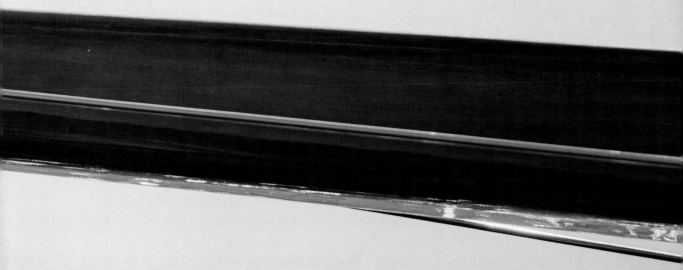

STERLING
New York

An Imprint of Sterling Publishing, Co., Inc.
1166 Avenue of the Americas
New York, NY 10016

ISBN 978-1-4549-2813-3

Distributed in Canada by
Sterling Publishing Co., Inc.
c/o Canadian Manda Group, 664 Annette Street
Toronto, Ontario, M6S 2C8, Canada

For information about custom editions, special sales, and premium and corporate purchases, please contact Sterling Special Sales at 800-805-5489 or specialsales@sterlingpublishing.com.

Manufactured in China

10 9 8 7 6 5 4 3 2 1

sterlingpublishing.com

A complete list of photo credits appears on page 223.

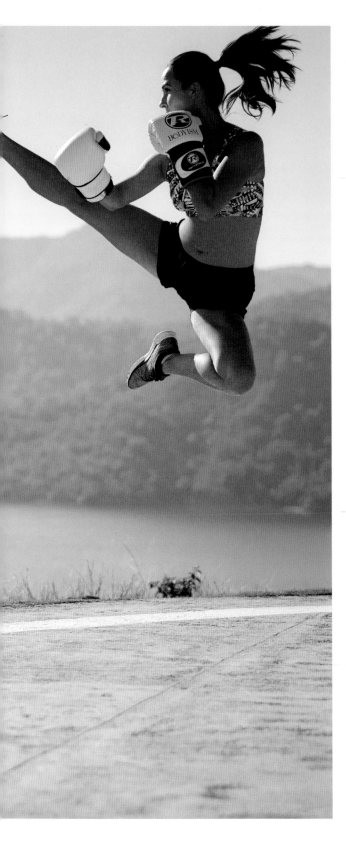

CONTENTS

THE PILLARS

8   Author's Note

10   Introduction

12   Ⅰ Mindset

24   Ⅱ Nutrition

46   Ⅲ Movement

74   Ⅳ Sleep

88   Bodyism Two-Week Plan

THE RECIPES

94   Breakfast

118   Lunch

140   Dinner

170   Snacks and Sides

192   Desserts

214   Bodyism Basics

222   Index

224   Final Thoughts

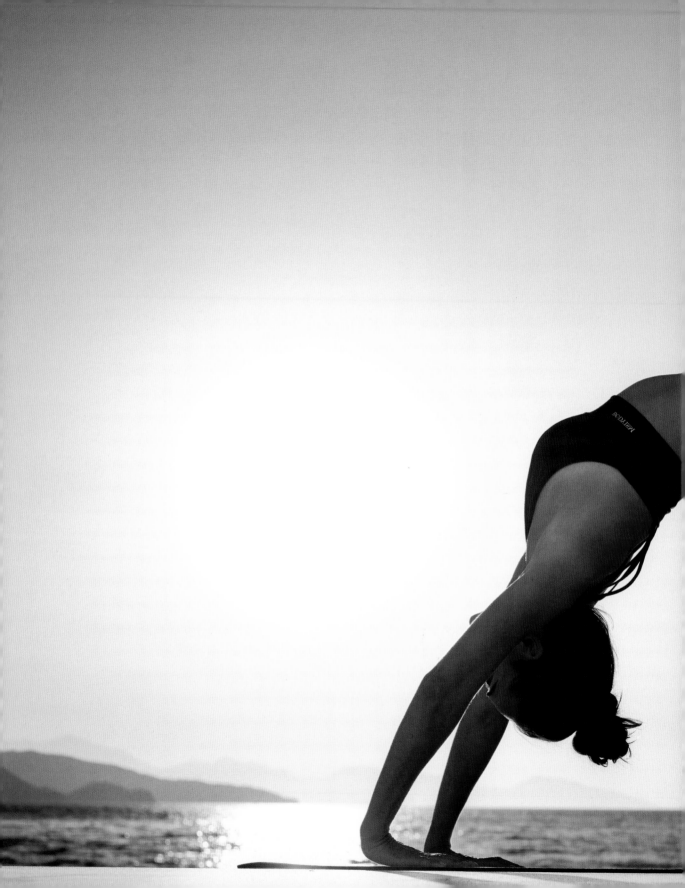

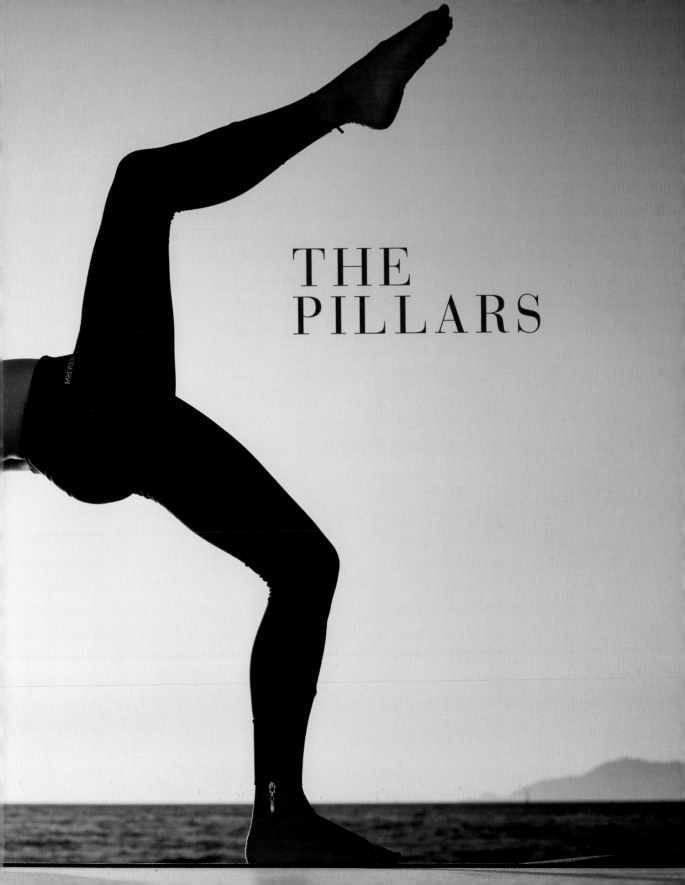

THE PILLARS

AUTHOR'S NOTE

"Be open to everything, to all possibilities, listen and be curious." —DR. WAYNE DYER

Mindset, nutrition, movement, and sleep form the four key pillars of health. But living by these four pillars has never been more difficult to maintain. We have more ways to communicate than ever before, but we've never felt lonelier. More food is being mass-produced, but we've never been more malnourished. There is more research about the importance of sleep than ever before, but we've never been more sleep-deprived. Gyms are popping up on every corner, but we've never been less active. The Bodyism® ethos follows the simple philosophy: Be kind to yourself. No superfood, health trend, or exercise class can do that for you, but by making positive changes to each of the four pillars of your health, you can.

This is a really momentous point in my life because, as I write this book, I feel that I have finally found balance across all four pillars of health. If you don't feel balanced, I understand. I've been there. Over the years, even while writing bestselling books, running the most luxurious gym in the world, and standing at the forefront of the wellness industry, I still struggled to come to grips with each of the four pillars. So don't beat yourself up, just return to our simple philosophy. This book will show you how to navigate today's world so you feel and look healthy, achieve your optimum state of wellness, and truly learn to be kind to yourself.

Throughout this book (and for the rest of your life), look at the four pillars of health equally. See them like the tires on a car. As you travel through your life, if one of those tires misaligns or fails, eventually, it will cause some problems. The more out of alignment that tire is, the more serious these issues become

and the more quickly they will impact one another. Just as a mechanic pays equal attention to each tire, we need to pay the same amount of attention to each pillar of health. When we make positive changes to each pillar, our overall sense of wellness will improve. It's time to change your life.

First, you need ask the right questions.

Why don't diets work? Why do so many people fail in their pursuit of health? In large part, people are looking for answers when they really need the right questions. Always start with your "why." "Why do I want to lose weight?" "Why do I want to eat well?" "Why do I want to feel healthy?" My "why" is "Why do I want to live a long, healthy, and happy life?" My answer is "To be a strong father for my kids and one day grandkids." That "why" keeps me focused on making the right decisions with all four pillars of health.

You're looking at this book, so you're already halfway there. You already want to make a change. You probably know why you want to make that change, and now you're trying to figure out how to do it. My *Blueprint for Health* will offer questions and answers to help you understand the importance of the four pillars and your connection to them.

A word of warning: my intention is always to help. I want to be truthful. I don't want the message to get lost in diplomatic fluff. Choose not to be offended. Being offended is a waste of time. Take inspiration from Dr. Wayne Dyer and choose to be curious.

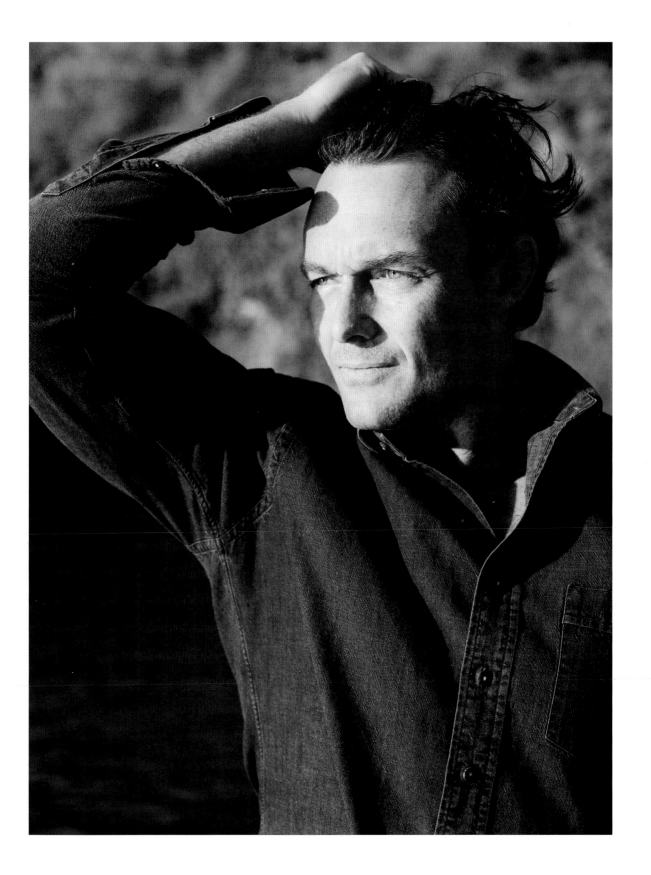

INTRODUCTION

Nutrition: Beware of cat

My understanding of the four pillars began early in life. When I was five years old, I was hyperactive and had behavioral problems. I literally couldn't sit still, I was constantly in trouble at school, I couldn't sleep through the night, and I remember not feeling comfortable in my own skin. My parents took me to a doctor, who prescribed sedatives throughout the day to "control" my behavior, tranquilizers at night to "help" me sleep, and steroids to "fix" my cough.

Even back then (35 years ago), my parents felt that was a heavy amount of drugs; it seemed like a hell of a lot to put a tiny kid through.

Somehow, they managed to find a naturopath, Helen Neitzsche. She said: "Why don't we take him off sugar for a couple of weeks and see how that goes?" I wasn't eating anything out of the ordinary; I followed a "normal" diet: sugary breakfast cereal with a glass of orange juice in the morning; a chocolate doughnut at morning recess; maybe a sandwich at lunch. Back home I had some chocolate milk; dinner usually consisted of a pre-made oven meal. (Only super-fancy people had microwaves.) Then, for dessert, a bowl of ice cream with chocolate sauce. Looking back, this was a horrendous amount of sugar, but parents back then didn't know what they do now. That you're reading this book means that you have at least some interest in health and wellness, but many people would look at that diet and think it was absolutely fine—and yet wonder why they or their family were suffering from poor health.

My parents followed the naturopath's advice and cut my sugar intake. After three days, I was behaving like a normal person. I remember suddenly feeling calm rather than "wired and tired," as I had felt constantly when I was high on sugar. At the end of that first week, our pet cat ran away, and my cough instantly disappeared. Turns out I was allergic to cats. If it wasn't for the doubt of my parents or a cat yearning for freedom, I could have been on the road to a drugged-up life of sugar addiction, chemical addiction, and illness. So, early on, I understood the powerful connection between what you eat and how you feel. That's how I identified the pillar of Nutrition.

Movement: Getting fat

When I was eight years old, I went to live in Flying Fish Point, Queensland, Australia. I barely went to school; I spent my days chasing butterflies, fishing, climbing trees, and making stuff with whatever I could find in the rainforest. I picked fresh papayas, mangoes, and avocados off the trees. (Health tip: eating anything freshly picked is one of the best things you'll ever do for your health and is one of the most powerful sources of probiotics you can get.) I was so active, healthy, and happy. Then I moved with my mother to Barnsley, in the north of England and had culture shock. I spent my days watching *Dallas* and *Dynasty,* and I slipped back into a toxic, high-sugar diet. I felt awful and I got fat.

The first time I had any inkling that I had changed was when I returned to Australia. My dad hadn't seen me for months. He opened the door and said, "Bloody hell! What happened to you? You got fat." He said it straight: "Come on, mate, you need to sort it out." My dad was the most gentle and loving person in the world. I'm sure what he said sounds harsh and, coming from anyone else it would have been, but he was such a gentle soul, and he knew how to speak the truth. I didn't wait one minute. I put my bags down, tied the laces on my boots, and ran around the block. That was the first time I realized how amazing the simple act of moving made me feel. I didn't wait even an hour to go on that run, I recognized the power of now and felt excited. That was the day I realized what a powerful effect movement has on how you feel and how you look, too. That's how I identified the pillar of Movement.

Mindset: Night buses

In my early twenties, I went to London with fifty dollars and no plan. I look back on it now and wonder what the hell I was thinking. As we were landing, I remember turning to the person sitting next to me on the plane and asking her where I should stay. I genuinely had no idea what I was doing, and, sure enough, within about two weeks, I was homeless.

I probably could have asked for help, but I was too proud. I was sleeping on night buses and eating food from the bins outside Starbucks. I bought a suit and a pair of shoes from a thrift store (the shoes wore out within a week, and I patched them up with cardboard) and I managed to get myself a job at Harrods. I lived a double life for about eight weeks; I was working in one of the fanciest department stores on Earth during the day while sleeping rough at night.

That was my rock bottom. Some people have had worse rock bottoms and other people never get as low as being homeless. Experiencing that low was quite liberating. My choices were very clear-cut—either I survived, or I didn't, I ate or went hungry. I chose to let nothing get in the way of my survival. I used that positive mentality, and it has stuck with me ever since. Rather than complaining or sitting and wallowing, I determined to succeed. That positivity has made all the difference. **That's how I identified the pillar of Mindset.**

Sleep: Tired of being tired

In my early thirties, I was working unhealthy hours as a personal trainer. I was constantly exhausted. If anyone ever asked how I was, my default reponse was "I'm tired," I said that so many times that it started to define me. I was a tired person. My friend noticed and said I needed to sort it out because I was going against the advice I was giving my clients. (That's why I always have compassion for people. It's so easy for these unhealthy behaviors to sneak up on us without us even realizing it.) I had become a "very tired person" because (a) I wasn't sleeping and (b) I'd convinced myself of it by repeating it over and over again. So I stopped telling people I was tired and I started making a commitment to sleep. It was way more difficult than I ever had imagined. Not sleeping had become an addiction. Solving this lack of sleep wasn't just a question of going to bed earlier, I needed to change my behavioral patterns and my mindset, and it took some work. I experienced that terror of not being able to sleep. I used to stay up until I was exhausted just so I didn't have to experience that "I can't sleep" feeling. Over time, I worked at it. I researched and read, and I learned new rituals, which prepared my body and mind ready for sleep. It improved everything: my productivity, my happiness, my physical wellbeing, my relationships, and it led to better decisions, both at work and at home. It completely transformed how I felt physically and mentally. **That's how I identified the pillar of Sleep.**

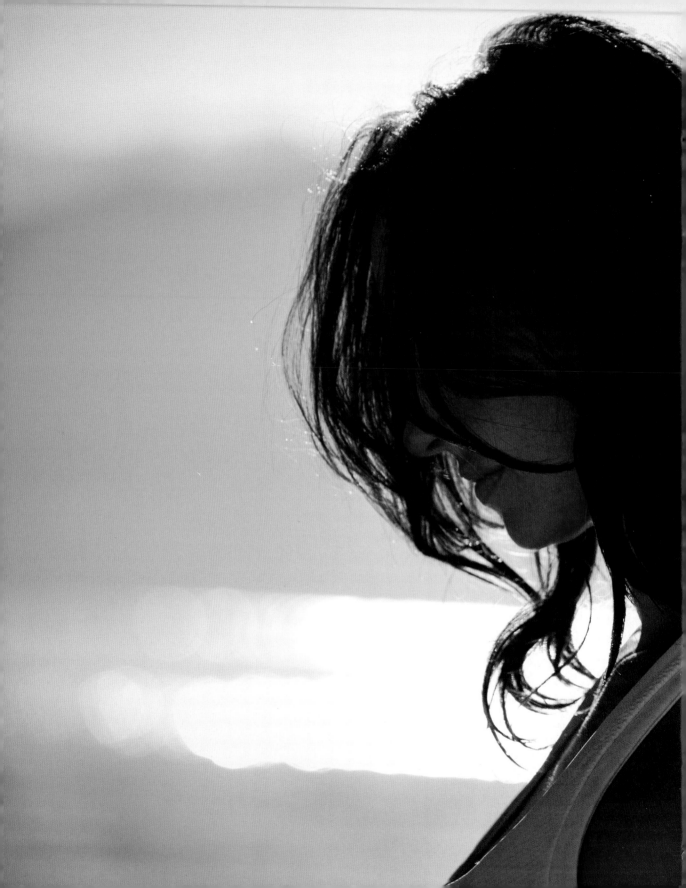

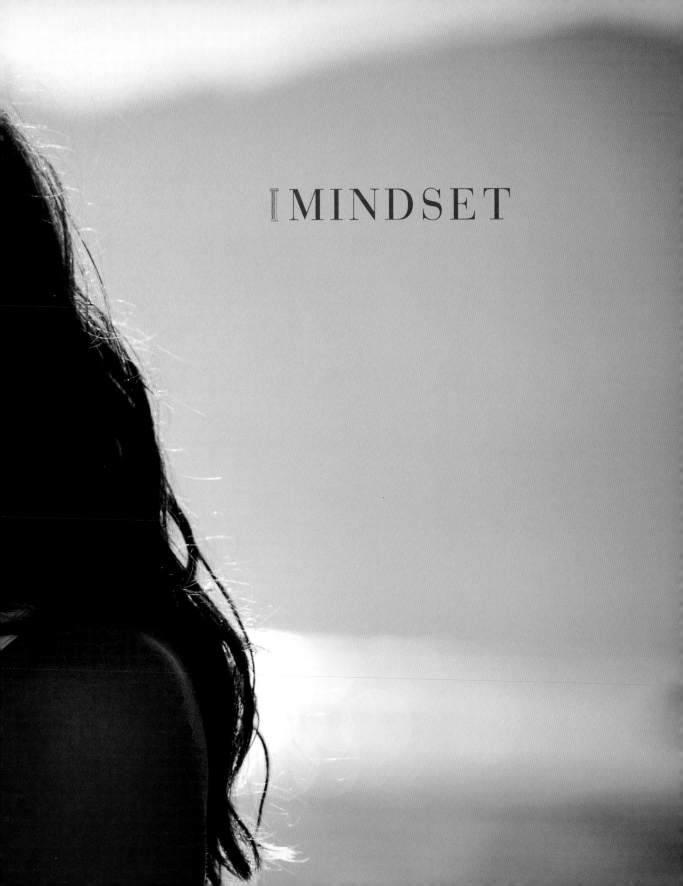

MINDSET

Why is mindset a pillar of health?

Mindset is such an under-appreciated and under-acknowledged aspect of wellness. How do you get your body into shape? You exercise. How do you maintain your physical transformation? You do it consistently, diligently, intelligently—and you stick to it. It's the same with mental health. I firmly believe that, just as we can use nutrition and exercise to help prevent poor physical health, we can take manageable steps to get our minds in the best possible shape, with the goal of living a long, happy, healthy life.

There's a lot of talk these days about mindfulness, but it's not just about doing yoga or downloading meditation apps (although there are some very good apps available, which I love). It's so much more than that. Yoga and meditation are simply gateways to learning the skills you need to attain mastery of your thoughts. Both will help you achieve optimum mental wellness, but you then need to incorporate the skills into your daily life, not just for the hour at yoga class or the ten minutes spent meditating. For mindfulness to work effectively, it needs to become part of the fabric of your life.

My wife, Christiane, made me realize the importance of mindset. When I first met her, I couldn't believe someone could be so truly happy. I was constantly scratching at the surface to see what was underneath. I realized that she was a genuinely positive and happy person, and once I'd seen that it was possible for Christiane (someone that I loved and trusted), I realized that it was possible for me, too. Because of how my mind works, I started to analyze her ability to be always positive, and I realized that we can teach ourselves to feel this way. Just like physical exercise, we need to exercise our minds, too—each is as important as the other.

Any change that happens in the body happens in the mind first.

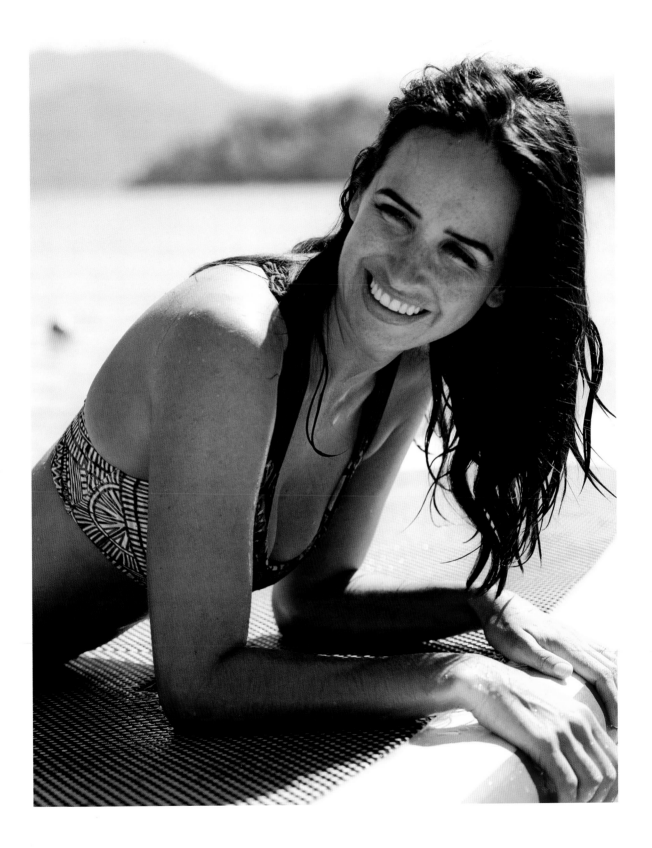

What does "mindset" really mean?

Mindset means the mastery of your thoughts. I often used to experience a phenomenon in which I had a sudden feeling of dread or disappointment in the pit of my stomach, which then hung over me for the rest of the day, week, or sometimes even the month. I have learned to stop this from happening by investigating the feelings further before they take over my entire being and cause unnecessary stress. I pause and ask myself, *Why am I feeling this way?* Then I search back through my mind and thoughts to work out what triggered it. I have come to understand that this sudden multitude of low feelings is caused by a negative situation, thought, or memory that usually can be dealt with easily once I recognize it. Had I been aware of it at the time, I immediately could have addressed it, rationalized it, resolved it or, at the very least, made a conscious decision either to let it go or deal with it rather than ending up with a constant hum at the back of my mind, dictating how I feel. Mindset is the process of investigating negative feelings and learning to focus on positive thoughts. Allow your mindset to help master your thoughts.

What is the perfect body?

The perfect body is one in which you feel happy and healthy. Plenty of people in the public eye, despite having a low body-fat percentage and posting endless enviable "selfies" online, are, in fact, constantly miserable. You can't have a "perfect" body if you don't have a healthy mind. One of our Bodyism mantras is, "Any change that happens in your body must happen in your mind first." The key word here is "first." Your thoughts determine what you choose to eat, how often you move your body, and the amount of rest you give yourself. So your commitment to being healthy comes from how much you love and accept yourself.

Too many people obsess over how they look. They allow it to consume every aspect of their lives, which is far from healthy. There's often a "when"

mentality: when I am skinnier/more toned/have a flatter stomach—then I'll be happy. I've worked with supermodels and well-known actors for many years, and I can promise you that the validation they are seeking (that we all are seeking) from other people will never be enough. It doesn't matter what you're seeking, be it a compliment from a friend or significant other, appearing on the cover of a magazine, or winning an award for being "the world's most beautiful." I guarantee you, it will never be enough.

We all suffer the same insecurities, self-doubt, and fear of lacking. It takes a huge amount of strength and self-discipline to get yourself off the misery train to crazy town. You need to value yourself beyond your weight or body-fat percentage. You need to value yourself for your kindness, talent, ideas, and integrity, and only then will you begin to see a shift in your life as you finally start to experience happiness. That elusive "when" finally will become "now." With the right mindset, you can embrace the power of now. The perfect body is more about feeling mentally positive than anything else.

What are affirmations?

Affirmations are positive statements that define you as you want to be. Affirmations help make goals feel real. If you look back through history, in every era and culture, when people want to find strength, they speak to a higher power—whether it's God, Buddha, Allah, Simon Cowell, whoever. To say something aloud gives it power. Choose your words wisely and use them kindly. The universe will listen to what you are saying; I truly believe that.

Chrissy and I have learned from people far wiser than ourselves that the way you frame affirmations really matters. We phrase them as if what we want already exists and we are already grateful for it. When you're grateful, it means something good has happened in your life, so feeling gratitude is one of the most positive and powerful states of being. You might say: "Thank you for my healthy body." You may not have reached optimum health just yet, but speaking of it as if it already exists, with no question or room for failure, makes it feel so much more achievable.

Here are some other examples you might try:

Thank you for my happy life.
Thank you for my wonderful partner.
Thank you for my comfortable home.
Thank you for my nutritious food.
Thank you for my gold tooth.

The last one's a joke, but whatever you have committed to bringing into your life, speak of it as if it already has happened, as if you already are grateful for it, and then imagine how it would feel to have it in your life. The power of affirmations is real and you can experience the incredible effects of using them.

A lot of cynicism surrounds affirmations. Those who doubt their power don't get it. People would rather be right than happy. Let me explain.

Take, for example, people who say, "Everyone will screw you over." With a strong negative view like this, they will find themselves drawn toward people who *will* screw them over, or they may create a situation in which they receive poor treatment so they can prove themselves right about what they so firmly believe and have told themselves over and over again. Whatever it might be, the more you say it, the more "right" you will be about it.

How can I make my mind positive?

I often tell my clients about a Cherokee legend called "The Two Wolves," which clearly demonstrates the mastery we can achieve over our minds.

An elder Cherokee is teaching his grandson about life. "A fight is going on inside me," he says to the boy. "It is a terrible fight, and it is between two wolves. One is evil—he is anger, envy, sorrow, regret, greed, arrogance, self-pity, guilt, resentment, inferiority, lies, false pride, superiority, and ego. The other is good—he is joy, peace, love, hope, serenity, humility, kindness, benevolence, empathy, generosity, truth, and compassion. The same fight is going on inside you and inside every other person, too."

The grandson thinks about it for a minute and then asks his grandfather, "Which wolf will win?"

The old Cherokee replies, "The one you feed."

Our thoughts can be our own worst enemy if we let them. Think about the negative stories that might be running in your mind. Many people believe they don't deserve a happy, healthy life—but that's not true. You may tell yourself that you're not good enough, too stupid, too ugly, or any number of other things that are totally untrue. These unhelpful thoughts don't have any purpose other than to reinforce habits that aren't constructive in any way at all. You've got to let all this stuff go because indulging in self-pity doesn't get you anywhere. You have the power to change the story running in your head. Once you're aware of it, you can let the negative messages go.

One of my clients used to think, *In order to be seen to be working hard, I have to seem stressed and unhappy. I can't show any joy because then it looks like I'm not doing my job.* During our training sessions. I started to notice evidence of this mindset. I asked if she liked her job, and she said she really did. I suggested that people still would think her a hard worker even if she smiled. She quickly became aware of the negative story running in her head, and her general level of happiness increased, as did her productivity at work.

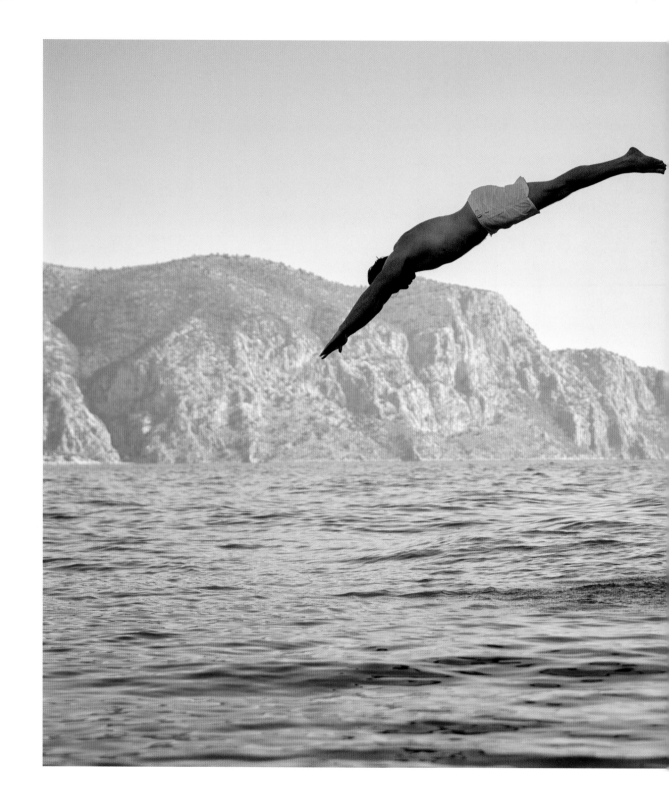

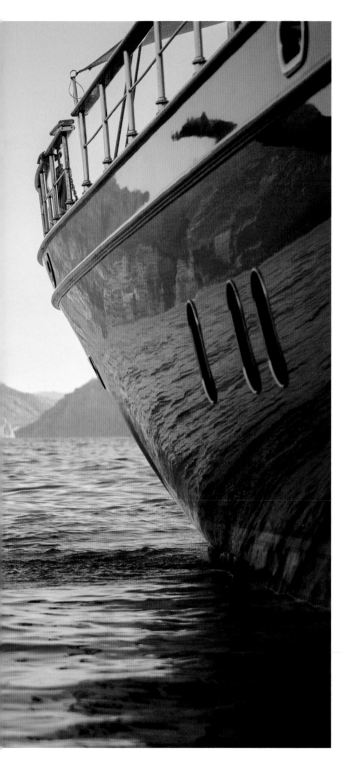

Similarly, I was at a party, chatting with a friend who works in the music industry. He wanted to talk to someone whom he really admired but couldn't pluck up the courage. I asked why he wouldn't just go and introduce himself, especially since meeting this guy had the potential to improve his career. His response: "I'm just shy."

I asked "What makes you shy? Is there a shy gene? A shy cell? A shy hormone?"

For the first time, he stopped and thought about it and eventually said, "No, there isn't a reason. Maybe I'm not shy, it's just something I've been telling myself."

That's a very powerful example of someone running a story in his head that created a false construct of reality. You have the power to change your story, so make it a positive one. You can invent whatever you like about yourself. Tell yourself you're confident, loving, and capable of doing incredible things in this world. Change your story to that. Why not?

We all construct stories about ourselves in lots of different ways. It's not easy to step out of your internal comfort zone and really address these negative habits, but it is possible and can transform the way you experience the world. If you were overweight, you would look at your lifestyle and ask, "What am I eating?" or "How much am I exercising?" and then make changes. If you're emotionally unhappy, why wouldn't you ask yourself: "What do I generally think about?" "What often preoccupies me?" or "Where do I devote my mental energy?" In other words, which wolf do you feed? (Whichever wolf you choose to feed, try to make it gluten free!)

How can I be more positive?

Most of what we worry about and what makes us anxious, upset, stressed, and miserable isn't actually happening and never will. The philosopher Michel de Montaigne said it best: "My life has been full of terrible misfortunes most of which never happened."

So let your worries go because—remember—most of them will never happen. No more stressing about something at work, a judgmental look that someone gave you (probably while holding in a fart after eating a crappy lunch), or what someone else is thinking about you. It's important to know that everyone is just as self-obsessed as you are, and they're probably not thinking about you at all. Rather than getting caught up in negative thoughts, focus on the here and now.

Often, when I'm stressed or anxious, I will do the following self-reflection exercise to remind myself of what I am grateful for in that moment. I might say, "Right now, in this moment, I am safe and warm, I am fed and I am okay. In this moment. That is everything I've got."

This exercise has saved me in the past because being present has empowered me to make strong decisions and choices and has helped me navigate some troubled times.

If, in that same moment, you feel sad or low, don't resist it. Accept it and let it pass like a cloud over a blue sky.

How can I break a habit?

I have been working for twenty years with clients who are trying to give up a habit, such as smoking or drinking. Often they've been working with a hypnotist or some guru, which never works because the only person who can end your bad habits is you. No other person, pill, or magic spell can change your life—only you can change your life. The power lies within you.

I fall easily into habits, so I really do understand where people are coming from. I regularly slip back into bad habits before I even know it.

Here is an example of one of my (admittedly very lame) addictions . . .

For years, I frequently ate a big slice of gluten-free bread with loads of butter and hazelnut spread. I ate it every night before bed and that was my thing. It got to the point where I had fallen into a cycle of addiction; I couldn't *not* have it. I always felt gross the next day—I had a constant food hangover. I used to hear this voice in my head (the gluttonous voice of stupidity) which said: "I really feel like it" before starting to justify it even more with "I need it," and "One more night makes no difference" and "This is the last time." Probably more than three months passed before I ate it for the last "last" time. I could have gone on like that for the rest of my life.

This is possibly the nerdiest story of addiction ever told, and I'm almost embarrassed that I don't have a heavier story to share, but it doesn't matter what the addiction is; it's the same thing, the same voices justifying it. It doesn't have to be alcohol or drugs to make you an addict.

Finally, I had to admit to myself that I was addicted. My drug of choice was gluten-free bread and hazelnut spread, and, yes, I see the humor in this addiction story! It's frightening how easily you can talk yourself into things. That voice in your head is very persuasive, and you have to say, "I have to stop." I said no to the temptation, I shut the cupboard door, and I held tight. I had a relapse or two, but I got through it.

Remember, it's not just the substance you get addicted to—it's also the ritual. For me, it was the motion of putting the bread in the toaster, layering on the butter, lathering on the spread. It's the same for those who crave a glass of wine at night. The solution is to swap it for a healthy habit that fulfils the same function. Find a healthy ritual that fills the void. Instead of pouring a glass of wine, treat yourself to five minutes of yoga or relaxing breathing, a warm bath or a cup of tea. Does that sound less satisfying? Maybe. Will it change your life? Definitely. Go for a walk, listen to some music. Find a healthy replacement for the bad habit.

There's no secret technique to doing this. If there were, a lot more people would be free from their bad habits, and significantly fewer people would be obese, unhealthy, and unhappy. There's no shame in being an addict. Many of us have that personality trait, gene, or chemical impulse, but you need to recognize that a particular habit is making you miserable and that it needs to stop. Ask yourself, "Why do I want to break my habit?" If you have a strong enough "why," it will carry you through the challenge of breaking any bad habit that might otherwise seem too difficult.

5 ways to stop late-night eating

One of the most difficult habits to break is late-night eating. Naturopath Rhaya Jordan shows us five ways to break the habit:

1. **Wear yourself out.** Most of us are too sedentary in the day (sitting at our desks, sitting for our commute, and sitting some more for lunch). Try to use up your physical energy within your day—even if that means getting up 30 minutes earlier to walk to the next bus stop or going on a quick walk during your lunch break or after dinner. Tire yourself out so you want to go to bed at a sensible hour.

2. **Fuel up.** So many people under-eat during the day and then make up for it at night. Think through your schedule logically. In the morning, you need to power yourself up with enough energy for the day, so have a wonderful, nourishing breakfast (pages 94–117). Then, rather than underfeeding yourself and dragging your metabolism down with you, eat when you're hungry during the day so that at night (after a nourishing dinner) you can let your body and mind wind down rather than stressing it out with unnecessary late grazing.

3. **Create a rest routine.** Sleep is nature's gift, so be thankful for it! Come up with rituals that help you wind down which will make you way happier and healthier than late-night snacking. Light a relaxing candle (remembering to blow it out before you go to sleep). Keep your bed looking comfy with big squishy pillows and a beautiful soft throw. Drink a cup of herbal tea or read a good book in bed. Reserve your bedroom just for sleep and sex, and take any stress out of there. When you start looking forward to bed, the temptation to eat might loosen its grip.

4. **Say it straight.** When your inner grazer starts tempting you into the kitchen, remind yourself that sleep deprivation is a huge factor in weight gain. It makes you put on weight, thickens your waist, and is just as fattening as alcohol. Be strict with yourself.

5. **Be a night gazer not a night grazer.** The end of the day is a wonderful time to reassess your goals. Write them down, watch a movie that gets you thinking, or chat with someone you care about. Switch off the TV food shows, which do nothing but wake up your dangerous grazer, and do something that you'll be proud of in the morning.

How can I encourage my partner to develop a healthy mindset when I am already there?

The truth is you can't. The minute you try to fix someone, it's going to make them feel broken. But you can encourage them subtly with small changes. If you're doing the grocery shopping or the cooking, then make sure you invite your partner to eat nourishing meals with you. Rather than saying, "You need to go to the gym," suggest going for a walk together. Make it a fun activity that you do together.

Change comes through inspiration, by being shown how good something can make you feel. No one ever changed their mind by hearing they weren't good enough; they have to realize the benefits of change for themselves. Often, people might resist because their self-esteem is low, in which case telling them they're lazy or fat or that they need to do it, can prove counter-productive. You have to live your own life, make those changes for yourself, and hopefully your partner will be inspired, encouraged, motivated, and supported enough to do it with you.

How does my physical health affect my mental health?

I see the incredible effects of exercise every day in people who walk through the doors of my Bodyism gyms. Shy, introverted people enter with a general fog of unhappiness surrounding them, but then they get their bodies moving and blood pumping and they transform, not just physically but also—and more importantly—mentally. They begin to smile more, they start to glow, and they generally look and feel more confident and happy.

Moving your body can make you feel better. It changes you on a hormonal and physical level. You don't have to go crazy on a treadmill—in fact, you shouldn't. Just go for a walk or do some yoga. Whatever it is, simply moving your body will help you feel a natural high.

When you feel stressed, angry, or anxious, rather than stewing over it, go for a walk and get your body moving. Once, when I was in a dark place and things weren't going well, I called Chrissy, and she said, "Go for a surf, just for me." It was a ridiculous suggestion— we had so much to figure out, and I had people to call and emails to send—but I listened to her. I went for a surf, and, my entire life transformed. Everything that seemed insurmountable suddenly became solvable. All the complications became simple. It transported me to a place where I could see a way out. So I always say, if you're stressed or angry and don't know what to do, move your body and then reassess; it could make a world of difference in realizing what you need to do.

What does it mean to be kind to yourself?

One of the driving philosophies of Bodyism is "Be kind to yourself." We believe in this phrase so much that we had it carved in stone at the front of Bodyism, London.

Being kind to yourself means understanding that you deserve a happy, healthy life. Recognizing that you are good enough, that you are worth listening to, that you are worth loving. So many people feel worthless, undeserving, and unlovable—but you are none of those things. I don't know everything, but I know this for sure. Once you recognize that, all the choices you make become easy. The pursuit of health stops being a battle and becomes a joyful way of life that elevates your experience of the world. Let this philosophy guide you through every section of this book and every aspect of your life. As you work through the four pillars of health, make being kind to yourself your guiding principle.

How do you do that? By choosing foods that make you feel good; by choosing to think powerful, positive thoughts; by choosing to surround yourself with people who support, encourage, and empower you. Remind yourself that you deserve a long, happy, and healthy life. Reaffirm your strengths and change that negative inner conversation to a positive one. Recite positive affirmations to yourself, such as, "I am unstoppable" "I am a good friend" and "I am a powerful person." Focus on believing them—because, whichever story you tell yourself will come true. Make it real and live your happily ever after, not just your generally-unsatisfied-about-my-body-weight ever after. No fairytale ever ended that way.

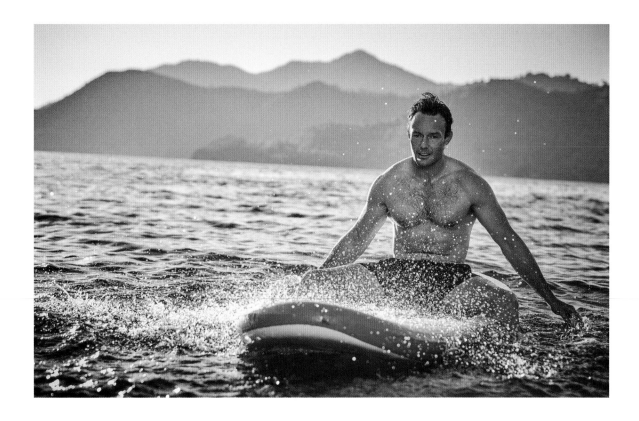

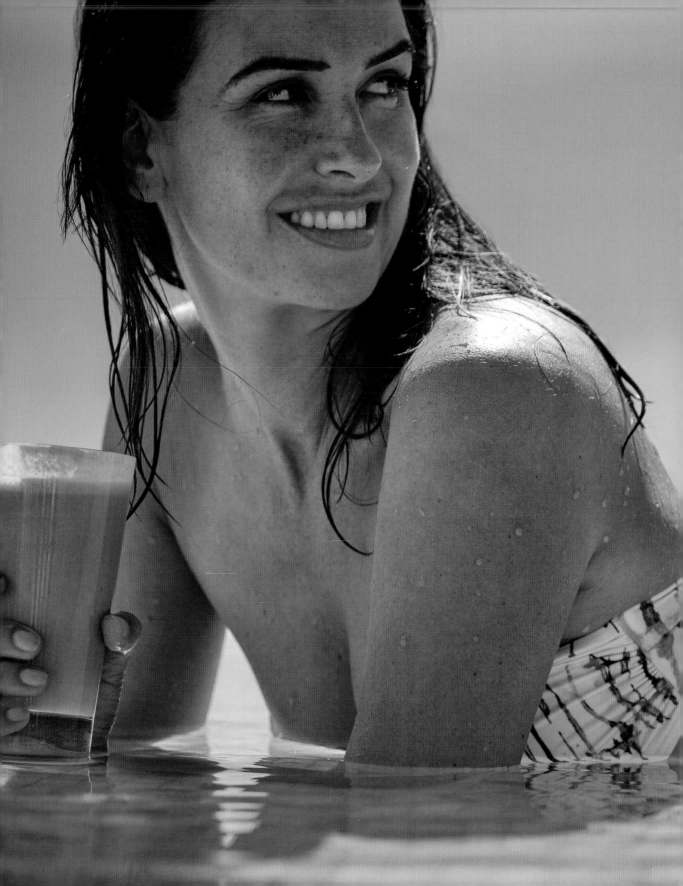

NUTRITION

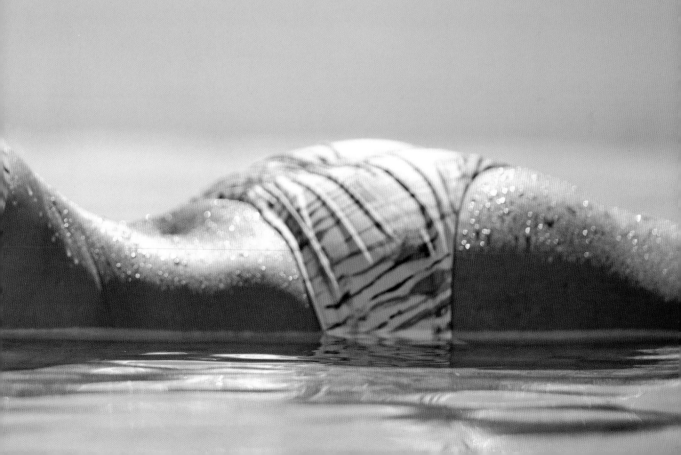

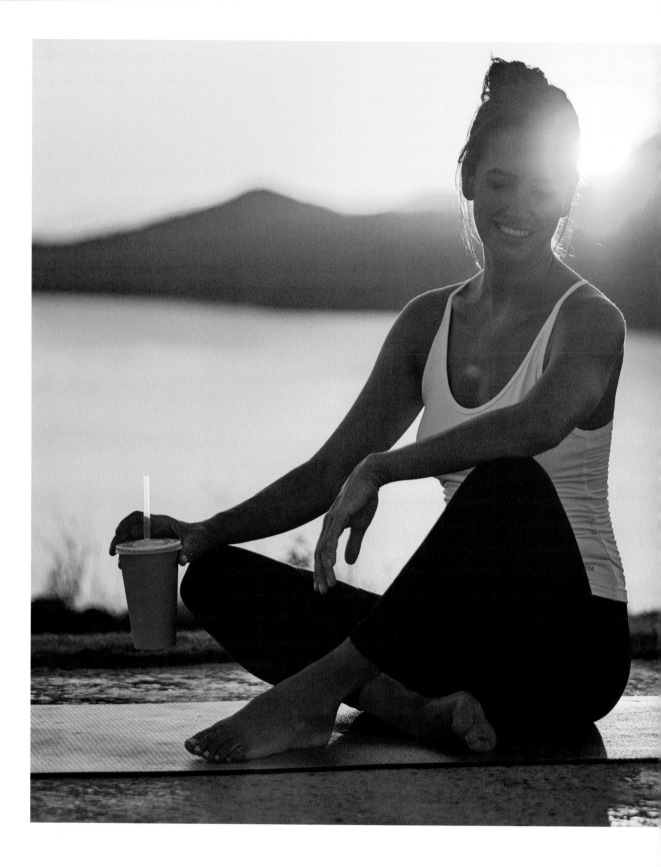

Diets don't work.

Why is nutrition a pillar of health?

Many people still haven't made the connection between what they eat and how they feel. They don't understand that nutrition is one of the four pillars of health. My goal in writing this chapter is to give you a deeper understanding of the effect that food has on how you look, how you feel, and even who you are. I also want you to be able to show this to loved ones so you can inspire change in them, too. What people eat today not only affects their health immediately but has long-term effects, too.

Over the years, people have asked me, "What's better to have in my water—lemon or lime?" "Which berry is best?" and "What's the exact amount of protein I should consume each day?" Don't worry about those kinds of small details. They distract from what you really need to be asking. You need to ask the bigger and more powerful questions that genuinely will make a positive impact. Questions like: "How am I feeling now, after eating that?" and "What am I going to do differently next time?" The answers all lie within ourselves. This chapter will shine a light on how to ask the right questions.

To help you find the answers, I asked Rhaya Jordan, a highly respected naturopath with whom we work at Bodyism, to share her expertise. Her knowledge will inspire you and equip you with a new-found understanding and passion for nutrition.

What does healthy eating mean?

People with the best intentions often do all the wrong things. In the early days clients came into Bodyism, saying, "My cholesterol is high; I need to stop eating whole eggs, and I can't have oily fish." We showed them the research that disproves that whole way of thinking. Everything I've been saying at Bodyism for more than fifteen years finally is becoming mainstream and widely accepted. But millions of people have died or suffered in the meantime, thinking they were doing the "right" thing. So it's time we knew which guidelines are truly healthy and what is, in fact, good for our health.

I don't know about you, but I'm so disillusioned and exhausted with all the different advice and diets out there. Which ones and whom should you trust? It's enough to drive even the most logical person insane.

Health no longer smells like lentils. It has become so much sexier and more superficial over the past few years, and therefore it's harder to navigate. Thirty years ago in a health-food store, the person working there was wearing a sweater made of leaves, had bloodshot, sleepy eyes and looked like they had wandered out of a commune—it was scary. I used to ask my mother, "Why are all the health-food people weird, and why do they look so sick?"

Health isn't weird anymore. It's mainstream, slick, and—for lack of a better word—cool. Wellness has become a powerful industry, which can be hugely positive if people are listening to the right messages. But when they're being sold something damaging, it can be scary and dangerous for their health. Only recently have people started to see through some of these health bloggers who have no life experience or professional qualifications and who are ruining this wonderful industry. Be aware of people dressing up their eating disorders with green juice; the truth is that they're just finding a different and more sophisticated way of saying "Obsess over your food," and it's giving others an excuse to justify such obsessions. This new flowery language of food empowerment often runs on nothing but shame and

guilt. Constantly asking yourself, "What am I going to eat?" "Did I eat too much?" or "Is it free from [insert almost everything here]?" is far worse than any diet. It's an eating disorder and it's got a name: orthorexia.

One Instagram user recommends eating 30 bananas per day. This isn't a fictitious example. That real person has thousands of followers and is ruining people's lives every day. Anyone who follows that person or other similar accounts and heeds advice to eat nothing but fruit has zero understanding of human biology. Our bodies just don't work like that.

I'll say it again: only balance works. The minute you begin to weigh your food, count your calories, or beat yourself up for going out for dinner, it's over. You're on yet another unsuccessful diet.

I wish I could provide you with healthy eating rules, but they don't work. Rules are made to be broken, and, more importantly, the human body doesn't respond well to rules. We're more complicated than that. Remember only one rule: be kind to yourself. That should drive every single choice you make. Beyond that, what works for one person won't work for another. So, rather than going on a restrictive banana diet, which isn't good for you and will plague you with shame, guilt, and gastro-intestinal distress, tune into your body and find foods that work for you. Your body will thank you for it and return to its natural state of "vibrant living."

How does mindset affect nutrition?

The Bodyism food philosophy isn't just about what you eat, it's also very much about how you think. How you think drives what you eat and how you feel. It's all interconnected, and each of the four pillars is equally important.

The energy you put into your food is almost as important as what you eat. If you have an unhealthy attitude toward food, return to the affirmations I mentioned in the mindset chapter (pages 12–23). Affirmations help with that mental struggle that so many people have. If I'm at home and bored, I tend to become psychologically starving, and that's when it's impossible to listen to my body. Rather than going straight to the fridge, take a moment and pause. Remind yourself of your affirmations: "I am eating to nourish myself," "I am grateful for this food." That moment of reminding yourself to be kind will make all the difference.

In the past, my attitude toward food has been unhealthy. I grew up hungry because we never had enough food. Even once I'd pulled my life together and knew where my next meal was coming from, that frightened eight-year-old inside me was telling me to eat everything I could. Here I was, pioneering an entirely new approach to food, health, and wellness, and yet I was still eating obsessively. I ate everything in sight until I was totally full. When I finally recognized the underlying beliefs that were driving my behavior and telling me I had to eat like that, I acknowledged that it wasn't working for me. Only then did it stop. It helped me kick that obsessive behavior and the untrue belief that food was scarce. Once I became aware of it, I could change it.

When you become aware of negative beliefs that drive negative behaviors, make a conscious effort to replace them with more positive beliefs. Doing so will significantly change the foods you choose and the way you eat.

When does healthy become unhealthy?

Chrissy and Nathalie (a trainer, Bodyism inspiration, and a total hero!) really taught me the importance of balance. I used to overeat "healthy" foods and constantly felt bloated and uncomfortable. I lived on nothing but green vegetables, fish, and meat; I felt guilty if I had any carbs and I always underperformed everything I did. I lived in a cycle of restriction and bingeing on cheat meals (page 41). Mentally, I'm strong, so I ignored how tired I felt. I grew accustomed to feeling dizzy: when I trained, in meetings, in general. On the outside, I looked fit and was eating a "healthy" diet. Now I recognize that I was being totally restrictive, and I was "gassed out."

Chrissy and Nat told me to bring abundance into my diet, to eat lots of colors, beans, brown rice, sweet potatoes, and fruit, and to have a more varied diet. So I did the Bodyism two-week plan (pages 88–91), stopped eating my cheat meal on the weekend, and that obsessive behavior quickly faded. I stopped beating myself up and took a leap of faith. I started to enjoy eating a more varied diet. The shame and guilt disappeared, and I really tuned in to how my body felt. When I finally started to eat a bit of everything, I began to *feel* energized rather than simply acting it. Today I look better than I've ever looked, and I've never felt happier and healthier.

The people on the edges are angry, boring, and unhealthy. Always remember that the middle ground is the safest, healthiest, and happiest place to be—it's fun here in the middle.

Rhaya Jordan: Feeling relaxed and flexible (mentally) are nice hallmarks of being healthy. When you feel angry at yourself for eating something "unhealthy," or if you can't concentrate on anything but your body or food, then that is stressful and not healthy. Here is the key, base your self-worth on the deep respect you have for yourself rather than what you see on the scales. If seeing that you've put on an extra pound ruins your day, you need to back off a bit and get some perspective. You deserve to be well—that's true health.

When I say, "Be kind to yourself," it's more than just a slogan or a cliché. What I mean is that you should let go of shame and guilt. Understand that your past doesn't equal your future; if you have failed before, use it as a lesson. Failure is feedback. Accept yourself so that you can create a powerful platform from which to move forward toward a happier, healthier you.

Are you still thinking about the Eiffel Tower? Now you are. That's why diets don't work.

Why don't diets work?

Diets depend on denial. If I tell you not to think of the Eiffel Tower, it instantly comes to mind. Similarly, if I say not to eat cake, most people reading this won't be able to stop thinking about it until their stupid diet ends and they can eat all of the cake—yes, all of it. What you resist persists. So rather than fighting your cravings and making it a battle, simply let it go.

What does this mean? The minute you make it a battle, it will have only one winner, and it won't be you. When you can relax, stop fighting, and understand that you

deserve to be happy and healthy, all of these battles become choices, and the choices become easy. The key is not focusing on what you can't have and instead thinking about what you can have. So often, health fads focus on giving things up, when they should tell you about enjoying amazing food that improves how you feel. Once you've experienced that, there's no going back. You might slip off the wagon, but nothing tastes as good as *healthy* feels. (Call me the Kate Moss of wellness!)

If you're choosing foods that work for you, make you feel good, and taste delicious, are you on a diet, or are you just living a happier, healthier, more intelligent life? Instead of going on a diet, how about deciding to be kind to yourself and completely changing your life?

Rhaya Jordan: Nutrition is a marathon, not a sprint. One of the best ways to look after your overall health is to change your behavior surrounding food, rather than signing up to another diet. Fundamentally, if you want to embark on real, deep change, you have to work *with* your body.

Ask yourself, "What food do I enjoy?" "What time of day am I hungry?" "Does gluten/dairy/sugar make me irritable or sleepy, or fill me with energy?"

Everyone is different and lots of these differences will be genetic, while some of them will be because of your gut microbiome (the natural bacteria in your digestive system). If you eat when you're hungry and stop when you're not, eat whole foods you enjoy and trust your body, you *will* get there.

Sometimes, people will need to do a "sprint"—maybe before a holiday in the sun or a big event—and, if that's the case, then try the Bodyism two-week plan (pages 88–91), which cuts out the main irritants for a fortnight and is a great way to refresh your system and work out what your gut likes and dislikes. But, if you eat poorly, then restrict, and then go back to eating poorly again, those extremes will cause more damage. The middle, balanced path is what's going to change your life forever.

What should I eat for breakfast?

What you have for breakfast will set up your body, psychology, and hormonal profile for the rest of the day. It also will determine what you crave throughout the day. If you start your day with sugar, you will find yourself on an all-day sugar rollercoaster. This is where the importance of sleep plays a key role (the final pillar, pages 74–87). If you don't have a good night's sleep, you're more likely to crave a quick sugar fix the next morning (more on this later).

We're all different, so there's no hard-and-fast rule for everyone. I'm what's called a "fast oxidizer," which means that I digest food very quickly. When I eat oatmeal for breakfast, it quickly spikes my blood sugar levels, and then I crash pretty quickly. Chrissy, on the other hand, is a slow oxidizer. She can eat pasta, oatmeal, or potatoes, digest them slowly, and they don't give her a sugar spike. She doesn't get the mood swings that I do, and her blood sugar levels don't dip and dive like mine. On the flip side, I can eat avocado, butter, eggs, and steak all in one sitting and, because I digest food so quickly, I don't end up feeling heavy; in fact, I feel energized—whereas a slow oxidizer would find that difficult for his or her body to handle. It's why the Bodyism coffee (Americano blended with coconut oil and butter) works well for me but is too heavy for some people. It's all about testing food to find the right breakfast for you.

As a general rule, it's important to start the day with some protein. You need it to nourish yourself and to feel full and energized throughout the morning. Day to day, it's all about listening to your body. One morning, you may crave lots of carbohydrates and energy, and you will feel great from eating that. On other mornings, you might feel more like a big helping of protein. Some mornings I wake up and crave avocado, eggs, and spinach cooked in butter, while other mornings I fancy a breakfast salad. Two years ago, if you had suggested the latter for breakfast, I would have stormed out. Now, I listen to my body.

It takes a while to understand what it means to "tune in" to your body, so while you're learning, I'll remind you of what doesn't work, and that's sugary breakfast cereals. These have almost no nutritional value at all, and a bowl for breakfast will make your blood sugar spike and have you craving sugar for the rest of the day. If you're reading this, thinking that you like your breakfast cereal, the reality is that you don't. You're addicted to the sugar hit. Try giving it up and having something different, such as half an avocado sliced up on oatcakes, or some oats, nuts, and seeds soaked in rice milk. If you're thinking, "Are you crazy?"—just try it; you might love it! It's so much better for you to eat a beautiful creamy avocado or crunchy oatcakes than a bowl of processed sugar and salt. Not to mention that ditching the toast and cereal sets you on your way to a flat, bloat-free stomach. Remember the quote at the start of the book: "Be open to everything, to all possibilities Listen and be curious."

Rhaya Jordan: Your first meal of the day should set you up for everything that follows, so make sure your breakfast is of high quality. An almond croissant to start your day will only send you spinning off on that sugar rollercoaster and you'll feel exhausted by lunchtime. There is so much new information coming out about our microbiome and how it affects the way we digest food. There are lots of different theories in terms of why we might find different combinations work well for us individually.

Of course, tuning in to your body has to be balanced with the demands of modern life. If you don't feel hungry till mid-morning, then just be prepared and, instead of going to your local convenience store and picking up something highly processed, spend ten minutes the night before preparing your bowl of oatmeal (Three-Grain Oatmeal, page 100), or keep some blueberries and almonds at work to enjoy when you are finally ready to eat. Try things out, find a pattern that fits your body and the end result will be much better. Appetite changes and varies, so tuning in to your body is the only answer. Intuitive eating is the Holy Grail.

Top Tip Start your day with food before your coffee (even if the food is a smoothie). Enjoy your coffee, but find balance and don't use it to replace breakfast (or to drive yourself when you're exhausted). The biggest problem with coffee is how easy it is to use it as a distraction from the real problem. If your coffee habit compensates for a lack of sleep and rest, then listen to your body and go to bed earlier instead of having a third or fourth cup.

What should I eat for breakfast if I have no time in the mornings?

1. **Smoothies.** Before you go to bed, put all of your whole ingredients in the blender, and then all you need to do in the morning is pour in the liquid and blend it up. That takes fewer than five minutes. See pages 216–219 for some great smoothie recipes.

2. **Jar prep.** It takes just five minutes before you go to bed to fill a jar with our Simply Granola (page 102). Add milk once you get to work, or make a Bircher Muesli (page 101), which you can leave overnight in the fridge and then throw in your bag and eat on the way.

3. **On-the-go.** You can buy pots of boiled eggs and spinach in most food stores nowadays, and, although less interesting than something home-made, they're ideal if you're struggling for time and will give you what you need to start the day off right.

4. **Go fish!** The British have a tradition of eating fish for breakfast. Pick up some sardines, kippers, and smoked haddock or even some shrimp if you can stomach it! Seafood is high in protein and a great option if you don't feel like eggs.

5. **Fruit 'n' nut.** If you're really stuck for time, grab a small tray of berries and some almonds—you can find those anywhere!

Rhaya Jordan: A smoothie is such a fast, easy, nutrient-packed meal. If you are rushing, it's a top choice, because the fact the food has been blended means it will be easier to digest and more soothing for your stressed-out digestive system. Please remember that smoothies you make at home are in a different league to the smoothies from a supermarket, which are normally higher in sugar than a fizzy drink. Smoothies in a supermarket shouldn't be called smoothies; they should be renamed liquid lollypops. Comparing homemade and store-bought smoothies is like comparing a Michelin-star noodle dish to a cup of instant noodles.

What should I eat when I'm out?

Enjoy your meal and don't amplify the damage or ruin it with feelings of shame and guilt. When choosing what to eat, think about what you genuinely will enjoy and what makes you feel happy not just in the short term but for the rest of the day or evening. Yes, it might bring you a sort of "pleasure" to have the bread basket and then a big plate of pasta and chocolate cake, but if it will make you feel miserable, lethargic, and bloated soon after, then maybe reassess which dishes you really want. If you're somewhere that has delicious fresh produce, like wild fish with seasonal vegetables, give it a go. You'll feel fantastic after eating it. (unless you're allergic to fish, of course). The trick is not to think about what you can't have but to focus on all the other amazing foods that you can.

How can I minimize damage from alcohol?

No one has to drink. People who say they have to drink – because of their job or for whatever reason – are kidding themselves. It's just not true. When clients tell me this, I simply don't buy it. You always have a choice. I choose not to drink alcohol, and yet I live a full and happy life. Take responsibility for your own life and your own health. Other people can do it, so what's different about you? Those people value their health, and they still enjoy themselves responsibly and have a great work-life balance. Remind yourself of your "why" before you make a decision (as I said before, mine is to live a long, happy, and healthy life) and let that influence you. If you really do want one drink, then have it, own it and move on from it. Remember, alcohol, by its nature, is a poison.

Rhaya Jordan: If you are going out somewhere to eat, go out and enjoy it! What makes the difference is your day-to-day intake, so a special one-off night out for dinner isn't something you should ever feel bad about. The French are a great inspiration, because they have the lowest obesity levels in the whole of Europe, despite the fact that they love cake. They enjoy food in small doses, lingering over their food, enjoying it mindfully, and eating it slowly. Also, remind yourself that you can have beautiful, indulgent food whenever you want; so, rather than eating everything in sight, remind yourself that you can come back and enjoy food like this again. This mindset will stop you from bingeing and purging (cake will always be around, so there's no need to eat it all up every time you go out). Eating out only starts to be a problem when you do it most nights, and that is when you might want more guidance. If your goal is weight loss, lean heavily on vegetables and go for protein, as it tends to help you avoid extra hidden sugars. Salads are always a good option, as are soups.

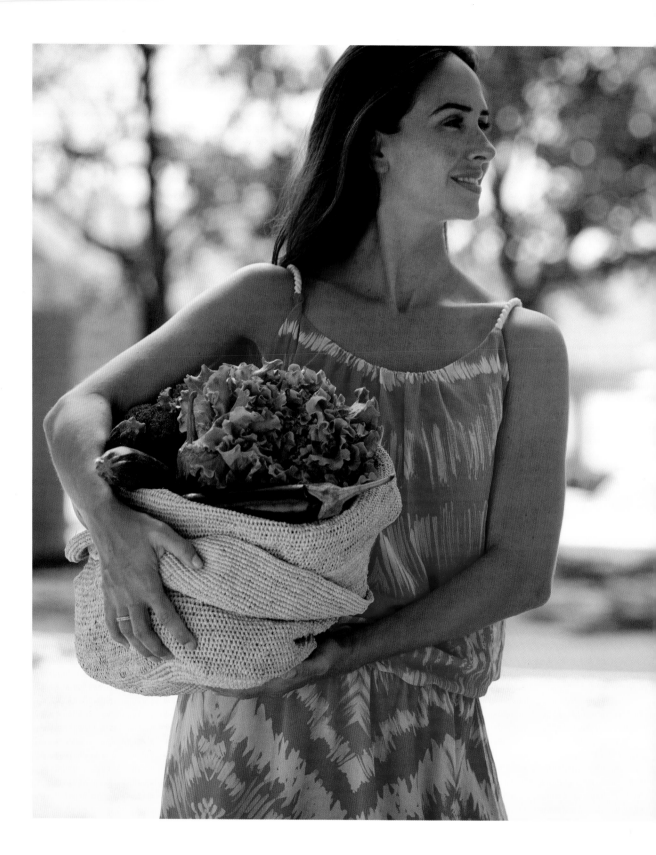

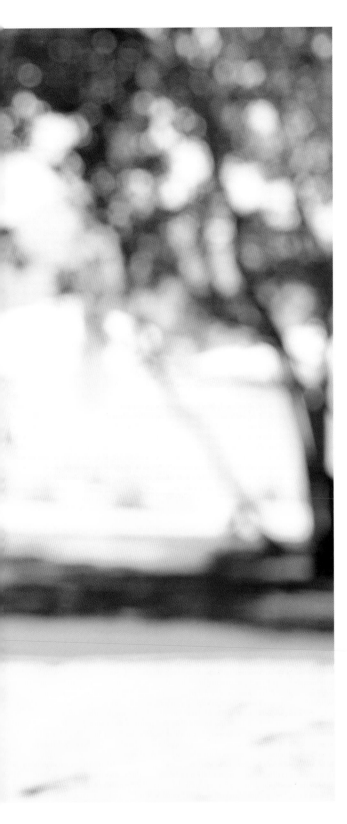

Rhaya Jordan: Alcohol is a carbohydrate, a simple one, and it does a lot of damage to your gut, your brain and your liver. Most alcohol is sweetened with some form of sugar or syrup and, because our gut is trying to expel the alcohol as quickly as possible, the sugar in the cocktail or glass of wine is very quickly converted into fat. So, whether we like it or not, alcohol is fattening and, more importantly, is not good for you. You can't "limit" the damage from alcohol, but what you can do is slow down the rate of absorption by having a meal with your glass of wine (or cocktail, if you must). You will feel the effect of the alcohol less quickly (so you won't say or sing things you regret), but don't forget you will still be consuming the same amount, just more slowly. If you do decide to drink, my "tips" for alcohol are:

1. **Choose red wine.** It's the only alcohol that's associated with any good health outcomes. But still keep your intake low and try to stick to no more than two glasses of wine (and always consider it a treat rather than a necessity).

2. **Keep it clean.** The cocktail with the least amount of sugar is vodka and soda water. That's a much wiser choice than a White Russian! Remember: the sugar from cocktails converts to fat very quickly.

3. **The one cocktail.** If you' are desperate for a cocktail, go for a freshly made Bloody Mary, as the tomato juice will have some benefits—but please make sure it's not lined with sugar syrup.

4. **Green cocktails.** Some fancy bars are now offering green juices as a mixer for spirits. Obviously these are wonderful, minus the alcohol.

5. **Say, "Cheers!"** Celebration and delight are incredibly powerful tonics; so, if you are going to raise a glass of champagne, don't then stress yourself out with feelings of shame and guilt. Own it, trust yourself not to drink the whole bottle, enjoy the celebration, and then move on.

What should I eat when I have no time to cook?

First of all, it's important to make time to eat. Every now and then you may not be able to and I do get that, because that's the reality of life, but bear in mind that if you have time to scroll through Instagram, then you have time to eat. If you often end up eating on the go, you're not being kind to yourself, and you need to change that habit. Eating energizes us, making us strong and powerful, so respect yourself and make time for it.

It would be wonderful if we all could eat lightly steamed vegetables that we grew ourselves from organic seeds foraged on a trip to Peru and blessed by a monk. Most people's lives don't look anything like this. Instead, you may have to grab whatever's handy when you're at home or on the go, and that means making sure you create an environment that influences healthy habits and bulletproofs your life from unhealthy options.

When you make dinner, it's a great idea always to make extra. That way, when you don't have time to cook you've got something ready to go from the freezer.

On the weekend, I bake a big batch of chicken thighs with Italian herbs, lemon and ginger, or the Bodyism rub (The Only Rub You'll Ever Need, page 214). I'll have a few thighs for dinner with brown rice and steamed greens and then keep the rest in the fridge for a super-nourishing, delicious, high-protein snack throughout the week. (It's also better for you than what you can find in most restaurants.)

If you haven't had time to make anything in advance, use your knowledge of whole, unprocessed foods. If you're out and about, rather than reaching for fast food, buy some whole "real" foods: cold meats, hummus, nuts and vegetables. You can get all of these at most convenience stores.

Will carbs make me put on weight?

Let's keep it very simple. There are real carbs and there are trash carbs. Choose your carbs wisely.

REAL CARBS
oats • sweet potatoes • broccoli • squash • parsnips • rutabaga • brown rice • quinoa • rye • barley • spelt

TRASH CARBS
white flour • sugar • white bread • white pasta • store-bought granola

Rhaya Jordan: Carbs won't necessarily make you put on weight. In fact, the Okinawans have the greatest proportion of centenarians in the world, and they tend to be lean and slender despite the fact they eat a large amount of rice. If it was true that carbs were the "demon," then none of the world's healthiest populations would eat them . . . but they all do.

So here is the problem: when we think of "carbs," we think of refined, processed, rubbish carbs. Get rid of that image and instead choose beautiful wholegrains. Adding a portion of these grains into your meal can be really satisfying. As always, listen to your body. If you feel good after eating them, then you've found a really great way to make your body feel full and content (and you'll therefore snack less between meals). Of course, it comes back to that individuality again, because some people can eat oatmeal for breakfast and yet still feel hungry all day. In case you want to know the science, there's an enzyme in the body called "amylase," which helps you break down carbohydrates. The more amylase you have (which is determined by genetics), the more easily you digest carbs

Many people think if they cut out carbs, they will lose weight. This isn't a lifestyle goal; it's a "quick fix" which can leave your overall health (and metabolism) the worse for wear. If you have a carbohydrate sensitivity, that is different, but if you want to look and feel good for the long term, remind yourself of balance: eat carbs, observe how you feel, and alter portions accordingly.

Word of warning: bad carbs suit no one.

Is not eating sugar a trend?

Sugar can make you fat, sick and can lead to an early, otherwise preventable death, so cutting back on sugar definitely isn't a trend. Sugar converts to fat more quickly than fat itself because it raises insulin levels, which causes fat storage. Studies show that 40 percent of the sugar you eat converts straight to fat – and that's in a slim person. Sugar leaches vitamins from your body, and a body starved of vitamins is a hungry one. As I've always said, "low-fat" food and drinks teem with sugar, because food companies have substituted the fat for processed ingredients—so they may not contain fat, but they will still make you fat. Don't buy them.

Should you cut sugar out completely? It depends on who you are. Refined sugar can be a trigger food. It can give you a sugar rush and behaves like a drug. It becomes difficult for people to keep their equilibrium. Some people find sugar so addictive that one sliver of cake becomes 37.

I have to avoid refined sugar completely because I'm an addict. I'll convince myself that I *need* chocolate cake, that I deserve it, and then I'll eat it every day until, two months later, I end up in Las Vegas, lying in a pile of chocolate cake, wondering how I got there. So I know not to start down that slippery slope.

Instead, I enjoy natural sugars from fruit, but I also know when I've had enough. I've learned to listen to my body.

But what's the deal with all of these "pretend" sugars? Be aware of the cool kids who pretend to be your friend but really aren't, including coconut palm sugar, agave, brown rice syrup, maple syrup, honey, and dates. In the same way that getting slapped in the face feels marginally better than getting kicked in the head, they're not *quite* as terrible as refined sugar, but they still aren't good for you. It's not a magic solution, so please don't think, *I can have as much of this as I want*. They still affect your blood sugar levels, your hormonal profile, and your weight. You may find maple syrup or other unrefined sugars

don't hit you as hard as refined sugar, but if you have a sugar addiction, just steer clear.

It's also worth knowing that some people in the wellbeing industry, considered beacons of health, produce and promote "health snacks" that contain more sugar than a chocolate bar. Every now and then, a newspaper runs a scandalous story on it and a few people become aware of the reality, but the vast majority continue to buy these "healthy" snacks under the mistaken notion that they are good food choices. Just because they're wrapped in brown paper and labeled organic or gluten-free, that doesn't make them any more healthy or less fattening.

Rhaya Jordan: If sugar was rationed tomorrow and it wasn't in so many drinks as well as savory food, then we could relax about a dessert or a bit of homemade cake. Back in the 1950s, sugar wasn't an everyday staple—it was a treat. But the way the food industry works now is so back to front, and sugar finds its way into practically everything, distorting your brain signals and making you wander into an addictive relationship with it. I'm shocked by how much sugar is in processed foods—sauces, cereals, drinks, even cold meats! The list goes on and on, and it's all gone totally insane. In the same vein, we shouldn't go to the other extreme and feel guilty about eating fruit or a slice of cake from time to time. As always, the middle path is the healthy option.

Rhaya Jordan: Until you really start to nourish your digestion and care for your body, you might have no idea what your true personality or mood is. There are two main ways in which we tend to undermine our digestion:

1. How we eat. We are designed to digest food properly only when we are relaxed. Remember, we are mammals, and our four-legged friends would not sit down for a meal if a lion was around; they'd be getting out of the way. To put this in modern terms, eating "on the run" is a disaster, because it makes us miss out a key stage of digestion called the "cephalic" stage. If you have ever walked past delicious-smelling food and felt your mouth water, then you know what this stage is: it's when you release enzymes into saliva which help break down your food. When you miss this stage out, your food doesn't get broken down properly and you get more fermentation, bloating, and gas. One of the key characteristics of people who live long, healthy lives is that they sit down to eat their meals. Chewing really well makes an enormous difference to your overall health—it could be the one thing that can transform your gut.

2. What we eat. Our gut is populated by trillions of bacteria that have a symbiotic relationship with our body. Justin and Erica Sonnenburg explain it perfectly: "Our microbiome (the gut bacteria) contains 100 times more genes than our human genome, so in fact there is about 99 percent of associated genetic material that we have the potential to mold in ways that are beneficial to us."

Our gut biome has an enormous impact on our overall wellness. Also, the microbiome determines how much weight you put on from the food you eat. Put simply, a group of bacteria called "firmicutes" are associated with weight gain. They change the way your body absorbs your food, and they love refined carbohydrates (sugar), which means when you choose processed foods, you are creating the perfect environment for firmicutes to grow, which in turn encourages fat storage. On the other hand, the group of bacteria called "bacteroidetes" help you metabolize food and have also been linked to reducing the risk of obesity, as well as illnesses like Crohn's disease and cancer. They love fiber, so choosing vegetables and fermented foods will help you get more bacteroidetes in your gut.

How does my gut affect my health?

People are suffering unnecessary gut problems because they aren't nourishing their bodies and generally don't go to the bathroom enough. We're friends now, so I can say it: you should poop every day. One of the biggest-selling pharmaceutical products is laxatives. This has got to stop. Last year, the FDA warned that the side effects of laxatives include severe dehydration, kidney damage, and swelling of the legs and feet. The other option is to eat more leafy green vegetables and fibrous foods. We need to think more long term about how to improve our gut health. The connection between gut and brain is so strong that even physicians have begun referring to the gut as your "second brain." It's where your "gut instinct" comes from.

Do calories count?

On a psychological level, counting calories simply doesn't work because, as humans, we're not designed to eat by numbers. The minute you bring that kind of thinking into the way you eat, you take all the joy from it, and it turns into a slippery slope of obsessive behavior and control that can lead to eating disorders.

A lot of people don't know that not only does calorie counting not work, but it's often totally inaccurate. The calorie content of food changes constantly. To determine accurately the total number of calories from a given food, you have to take into account a ridiculous number of factors, including the following:

1. How boiling, steaming, baking, or slow-cooking the food changes its structure and chemistry

2. How much energy the body uses by digesting the food

3. The extent to which gut bacteria help human digestion and, conversely, the amount of energy they use during digestion

It will never be exact. Ever. So counting calories becomes a pointless losing battle.

Look at the calories in an avocado compared to a bag of candy. The avocado has more. That doesn't mean you should reach for the candy instead, though, does it? The sugar in the sweets converts to fat, which you store around your internal organs and your tummy, whereas the avocado contains essential fats, which can help speed up your metabolism and will keep you feeling fuller for longer.

When I started working as a personal trainer, I spent time working in one of the best gyms in Europe. They have an incredible measurement system that calculates how many calories you burn throughout a day. Then they design an eating and exercise plan that puts you in calorie deficit. Sounds amazing, right? It's completely garbage. Why? Because real life gets in the way. Tuesday might be Dennis's birthday, and you have to eat a cupcake, which throws off your entire day. On Wednesday, you might have to work late and can't go to the gym. It's great if you're a millionaire and don't have to "live" life, or you don't have a partner, children, job, or anything else like that. But for most of us, that isn't our reality and never will be.

That calorie-counting machine is, in terms of calorie analysis, the most sophisticated operation I've ever seen, but I had to ask: does it work? Are you getting results? It felt awkward to ask, and the answer was no; they had less than a 10 percent success rate for exactly the reason given above: life happens. You are a human being, not a computer. It's not data in, data out. You're an animal; you have emotions, and you live with other people who have emotions and thoughts and different intentions and agendas, which means life can come at you and put any plan on the back-burner. Calorie counting has an almost heroic failure rate. Rather than eating by numbers, go back to the basics and choose food that truly nourishes you because not all calories are equal. You will feel amazing and look amazing, too.

What does "listening to my body" really mean?

A lot of people don't know they're sick because they've never been healthy. They're not in tune with their bodies at all. So many people think it's normal to wake up feeling tired, miserable, achy, bloated, and gassy. That's not normal; it's just common. Normal is waking up feeling energized, happy, and recharged. Often people don't realize they have an issue with certain foods because they're so numb from a general feeling of poor health and unhappiness.

Here's a story I often tell . . . A woman wakes up every morning, has a bowl of cereal, dresses for work, and walks to the bus stop, where she headbutts the wall ten times before searching through her bag for a headache pill. It makes her feel a little better, but she's constantly looking for a more effective headache tablet. What does this woman really need? A better headache pill or to stop headbutting the wall?

Believe it or not, many of us are doing this in the way we think about what we eat—we have a behavior that's causing an issue, and so we search for a pill, person, or diet to change us. All we need to do is stop headbutting the wall! If you're eating low-fat yogurt, doughnuts, three gluten-free muffins a day, or pasta every night, you're headbutting the wall. Instead, follow my blueprint for health and choose foods that work for you.

It can be scary to realize that it's all in your own hands, that no one and nothing else can change this for you. It's all on you. But once you realize that, you really can change your life.

Next, you need to recognize how your body communicates with you. This includes gas—we're all friends, so let's say farts—tiredness, bad skin, moodiness, irritability, bloating, aches, pains, inflammation, and mild depression.

If this is your "normal," you need to change because, if you don't, you'll only get more sick. These symptoms are your body's way of communicating with you.

Look at what you eat and know that you'll feel the effect within a few hours. If you eat a low-nutrient, high-sugar, highly processed meal, you'll feel terrible within 30 minutes. As I've said before, you won't be able to recognize this if you're on a constant rollercoaster of eating toxic foods. So try the Bodyism two-week plan (pages 88–91) as an introduction and then, when you add more foods back in, check in with how your body is communicating with you. If one or more of those negative symptoms are happening, think about what

Rhaya Jordan: Listening to your body can be scary or unfamiliar at first, but essentially, if you can tune in to your body and eat only when you are hungry and stop when you are full, your health and appearance will transform.

I work with obese clients and many of them eat in a trance. They eat until the food runs out, not until their body tells them to stop. To feel and look "healthy," you need to flip that on its head. You need to stop when your body wants you to stop, not when the food runs out. It's not easy to do. One great way of starting this is to eat without your phone, laptop, or any other distraction nearby. Your body whispers to you all the time, and if you are too busy or distracted, you won't hear it. So, when you eat, concentrate on just that. Be curious about what your body is saying to you. If you can do this, your body will help bring you back to balance faster than anything. Everything you need to be well and to achieve a healthy weight is there in your hard-wiring; you just need to pay attention.

It's important to learn the difference between listening to your body and giving in to cravings. Cravings will leave you feeling a bit twitchy and desperate, and normally you can judge if it's a craving by the quality of the food that you are after. If you have a lot of cravings, make life easier and don't put yourself in harm's way. So, if you often crave chocolate, don't keep it in the house. Grease the track in the direction you want to go. When you feel satisfied and content after eating, that's when you've been listening to your body.

you've eaten and look at what may be causing the reaction. Common trigger foods include wheat, dairy, sugar, and highly processed foods.

Why should I choose organic?

That people even debate about whether organic is better is completely insane. Let's keep it very simple: we know that pesticides cause harm to human beings, so you tell me which is better, a fruit that has pesticides on it or a fruit that doesn't? We know that the hormones used in non-organic meat are harmful to humans. So which is better, meat with harmful hormones in it or organic meat that doesn't have hormones in it? It really is that simple. It's more expensive to buy organic meat, true, so I have it less often. If you can't find organic, talk to the butcher and find out where they source their meat, or find a local farmers' market and do your research.

A study reported by Menus of Change stated that, "In 1960, the total annual U.S. expenditures for food were estimated at $74 billion. This was roughly three times as much as the total expenditures that same year of $27 billion for healthcare. Fast-forward to 2013. U.S. citizens spent $1.42 trillion on food and $2.9 trillion on healthcare, flipping the ratio, with healthcare spending now twice that of food." Invest in your health now and save on your healthcare bill later in life.

Rhaya Jordan: I have one sentence for this: have your food unpolluted. If you really can't afford to buy everything organic, then please at least make meat, eggs, dairy and fish your priority.

What makes a food "healthy"?

An important factor in a food being healthy is your attitude toward it and how you're eating it. Rather than thinking about what's healthy and what's not, think about being kind to yourself. With that attitude, you'll gravitate naturally toward the food that works for you, energizes you, and helps you achieve that perfect body. What's the perfect body? Severely overweight or underweight people can be completely happy, but the medical reality is that they're not healthy. Others have a wonderfully healthy body but are riddled with shame and guilt, so they're unhappy with it. Your body becomes perfect when it's both healthy and happy.

What is a "cheat meal"?

I used to swear by cheat meals, and my definition is indulging in whatever you want. (For me, that would be a chocolate and peanut-butter cake.) The science suggests that, if you eat a super-strict "clean" diet all week long and then let off steam and indulge in one cheat meal, it ramps up your metabolism so you wake up leaner the next day. I'll admit, I was once a huge advocate of this and loved the idea. The reality, however, was that it became an obsession. Halfway through it, I started to feel like garbage, my teeth tingled, and I felt uncomfortable in my skin. It wasn't pleasurable at all, but I had a psychological dependence on it. I felt like it was part of my job to have my cheat meal.

Now I nourish myself by making sure everything I eat is a joy. I'm not strict any more because I really do live by the rule of being kind to myself. I choose foods that nourish me, make me feel good, and are delicious and abundant. Living by that philosophy, I don't feel the psychological need for a cheat meal and don't have to blow off steam because I'm happy with how

I eat, feel, and look. Eating during the week isn't something I have to endure until the joy of my cheat meal. I feel balanced because my diet has so much more abundance. I have real carbs with my meals, such as brown rice or beans, which I used to think was a treat. I had created a joyless cycle and was living a when life rather than a now life. I used to think, *I'll be happy when it's the weekend*, but now I think, *I'm happy right now*, because food needs to be celebrated.

Check your internal monologue. If your thoughts are saying, *I'll be happy when I lose weight*, or *I'll be happy when I get this job*, whatever it is, let that go and let yourself be happy now. Sometimes life gets in the way, but, if you can, make a conscious choice to be happy right now.

If you choose to be kind to yourself right now, that horrible cycle of denial and indulgence will end. It's truly better to live without restriction and instead choose foods that make you feel good every day.

Are supplements a waste of money?

The short, truthful, correct answer is no—unless they are, in which case don't waste your money. What does that mean? In the world of supplements, there's no such thing as a bargain. If you're buying fish oils on sale, they're not going to work. That's the truth. If you're buying protein powder in a ten-pound bucket decorated with lightning bolts and a picture of some guy with veins popping out of his muscles and eyeballs, it's probably going to be bad for you. Cheap supplements, almost without exception, are a waste of money. In the supplement world, you really do get what you pay for.

Good-quality, ethically sourced, well-researched supplements do have an essential place in the modern diet, and here's why: food quality today isn't what it was 500 or even 100 years ago because of farming methods since the end of the World War II. (It has become progressively worse since then.) The fertilizers and pesticides that we use force food to grow more quickly but with fewer nutrients. Soil quality has deteriorated rapidly and so have the

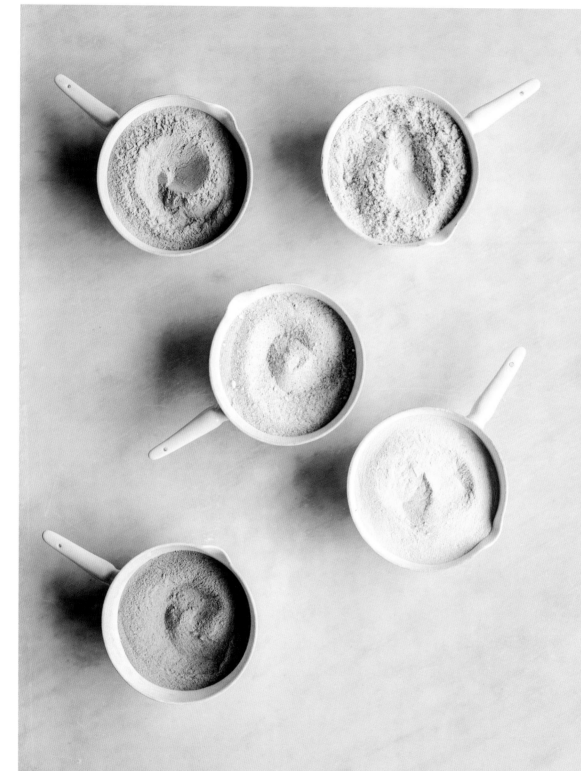

nutrient levels in our food. I wish I could say you can get all of the nutrients you need from the food that you eat, but I'd be lying. It's not the truth, and anyone who says so is probably living in a commune on an organic field—in which case, more power to you. If you've got a job and you live with the stress of paying your rent or mortgage and all of the other stuff that most of us face, then let's get real. Every now and then, you have to blend up a shake, drink it down, and be grateful for it.

People should take supplements to boost or nourish their bodies in an achievable way, where proper nutrition might otherwise be lacking for whatever reason. Because food quality isn't what it once was, we all need to supplement our diets. We also need a new word for them because nowadays supplements are essential. People need them.

As with everything, though, there's a balance. A medical professional once advised one of our trainers to take lots of vitamin D, so he did so and very soon felt really unwell. He had some tests done, which showed that he had toxic levels of vitamin D in his system. He was taking so many different supplements that he messed up his digestive system, suffered from erectile dysfunction, and lost his libido—all from too much of a good thing. You've got to be mindful and aware of what you're taking as well as how much.

What should I look for in a supplement?

There's so much dishonesty in the supplement industry, which is why, when I was creating the Bodyism supplements, I needed to make sure the products were trustworthy. I continue to make sure that the supplements are made fairly and that they actually contain the ingredients they claim to contain.

Rhaya Jordan: We burn through our nutrients faster when we are experiencing stress, modern pollution and lack of sleep. Supplements can bridge the gap in the modern world. A bad diet and supplements will not have a good outcome, but supplements can really turbo-charge a good diet.

Rhaya Jordan: It's a complete maze, so the simplest way to choose a supplement that is truly beneficial is to put a human you trust into the equation. Go to a health-food store and speak to someone who knows what they are doing. Look for some real food in the supplement's ingredient list (e.g. herbs, spices, berries etc.). The Bodyism supplements are the best I've ever seen.

With products like these, you need to have someone accountable put their name to them. We made each of our Bodyism supplements with a specific result in mind: to improve sleep, help you go to the bathroom, improve your skin, or improve libido. Supplements create a simple, time-effective, achievable way of getting everything you need to nourish you. Making a shake with supplements is a symptom of the modern world—not everyone has the time to grow a cucumber and sing to it.

A word of warning: if you're taking a really good-quality protein supplement and a supergreen mix, but then you combine it with a banana, mango, and pineapple, the sugar content of that smoothie is going to skyrocket. Be aware of what you're mixing your supplement with. Try almond milk or coconut milk, some greens (spinach or cucumber, not broccoli), and note the amount of sugar you're putting in there. It comes back to balance. Fruit is great for you, but in excess it's high in sugar, so be mindful—you can't eat 30 bananas and expect to be nourished.

Which ingredients should I avoid in a supplement?

Look for fillers, which are all extremely difficult to absorb and awful for you! These include hydrogenated oils, such as soybean oil, which is a source of trans fats; they're very cheap and absolutely terrible for you. Also watch out for talc, or magnesium silicate, and titanium dioxide.

Look for secret sugars, such as maltose, sucrose, and fructose.

Check the type of protein. Vegan protein (rice, hemp, and pea) is easiest to digest, so I always recommend that to my clients. Whey protein can work well, but it comes from cow's milk, so those with lactose intolerances may find it doesn't suit them.

See how you feel. As always, listen to your body. If the supplement makes you feel energized and recharged, then keep using it! If you feel bloated, change the portion size or try another supplement.

If you don't know an ingredient, look it up.

What should I do if I'm craving sugar?

Have a glass of water. I sound like a party pooper, but I'm not kidding because sometimes we crave sugar when really we're thirsty. Your body also might be saying that you need more protein, carbs, or fats in your meals. If you're under-eating or not choosing nourishing foods, you *will* be craving a sweet fix. Rather than reaching for a cheap sugar hit, have some nuts instead, some cold meat, or even a protein shake (chosen wisely). If you really want something sweet, go for fruit or bittersweet chocolate. If you can nourish yourself with some form of protein, you'll feel so much better than if you abuse your body with a highly processed, high-sugar snack.

What five "healthy" foods am I eating that could be making me sick?

1. Raw vegan energy balls. Check the sugar content. However they're dressed up, you could be consuming a huge amount of sugar without even realizing it. Try to find something genuinely healthy and nourishing because these balls can send you on a sugar-craving rollercoaster and result in a big sugar tantrum.

2. Smoothies from the supermarket. These can contain more sugar than a soda.

3. Green juices. Just because it's green doesn't mean it's vegetable-rich and freshly pressed. Just like some smoothies, some of these "green" juices contain about six apples and one spinach leaf. An apple is good for you but not a whole branch of them in one go. Check the ingredients carefully.

4. Low-fat yogurt. It tends to have loads of flavorings, thickeners, and a lot of sugar. Go for full-fat, plain yogurt with some blueberries instead of a fruit yogurt. Once again, remember that fat won't make you fat. It's more satisfying and will help curb your appetite.

5. Gluten-free food. Some of the "free from" products out there are processed, refined, super-expensive junk food. Gluten-free doesn't mean good for you. When someone holds up a gluten-free muffin as healthy, my heart sinks. Often producers have replaced the gluten with gums or upped the sugar content, neither of which is good for you.

What should I never eat after a workout?

1. A gluten-free muffin. No matter what it says, whether it contains refined sugar or pretend sugar, it's going to stop that fat-burning process within your body immediately. When you do cardio, you burn fat afterward until the second that sugar hits your mouth, at which point your insulin spikes immediately, which stops you burning fat. If you do a resistance circuit, you'll burn fat for up to three hours after you finish working out or until the second that sugar goes into your system. Instead, reach for a protein shake without a load of sugar in it.

2. Energy drinks. Especially the fluorescent ones. If you didn't already know, you never should drink anything fluorescent. These toxic drinks contain a chemical cocktail of toxic garbage. They spike your insulin levels, giving you a short-term sugar rush, which then puts you on that unhealthy rollercoaster of feeling wired and tired and will create, almost without exception, cravings and poor food choices for the rest of the day. Not to mention all the other funky stuff it does to your body.

3. Fruit smoothies. If your why for working out is to feel healthy and lose weight, don't sabotage your best intentions and undo all of your effort by consuming a load of sugar dressed up in a fruit smoothie. If it's crammed with pineapple or apple juice, it's not healthy. Store-bought smoothies look like your friends, but really they're the mean girls who want you to put on weight.

4. Chocolate cake. It may surprise you, but this is one of the most popular snacks that people buy at health clubs. In a study published in the May 2014 issue of *Marketing Letters*, people who were told that a one-mile walk was exercise ate 35 percent more chocolate dessert afterward than those who thought the same stroll was a scenic walk. The mentality is *I've just worked out, so now I'm going to reward myself with chocolate cake.* Now that you've learned the science about post-exercise sugar (point 1), you'll know better. You can't out-exercise an unhealthy diet; it doesn't work like that. Also, think about why you're reaching for the chocolate cake. If it's because you see chocolate as a reward and exercise as a punishment, then you need to change the story and find exercise that you enjoy.

5. Energy bars. Most of them are packed with natural sugars in the form of dates, which have an incredibly high glycemic-index load that not only stops the fat-burning process immediately but also contributes to weight gain. Athletes may require these short fixes from time to time, but, unless you're training professionally, these won't help you.

How do I know when I've eaten too much?

This is where listening to your body becomes so powerful. Rather than associating food with a fearful mind, eat with a calm, relaxed mind. When I was dealing with my obsessive behavior surrounding food, I repeated a mantra in my head before I ate: *I am safe. I am loved. I am in perfect health. I live in abundance.* (Don't say it out loud in public because apparently it "disturbs the other customers"!) Saying those affirmations helped me be mindful every time I ate.

Taking 30 seconds to tune in to how you feel before you eat and halfway through your meal can stop you from overeating. The easiest way to stop eating when you're satisfied, rather than over full, is to chew your food thoroughly. I notice customers eating at the café and it's striking to see the differences in how people do this. Some people eat so fast, with phones in hand, and it's a vacant, mindless experience. Sometimes, I'll sit next to them (not in a creepy way, promise) and ask, "How's the food?" What's surprising is that so many haven't even thought about the quality of what they're putting into their mouths. If this sounds like you, then work at it; it has the power to change your entire wellbeing.

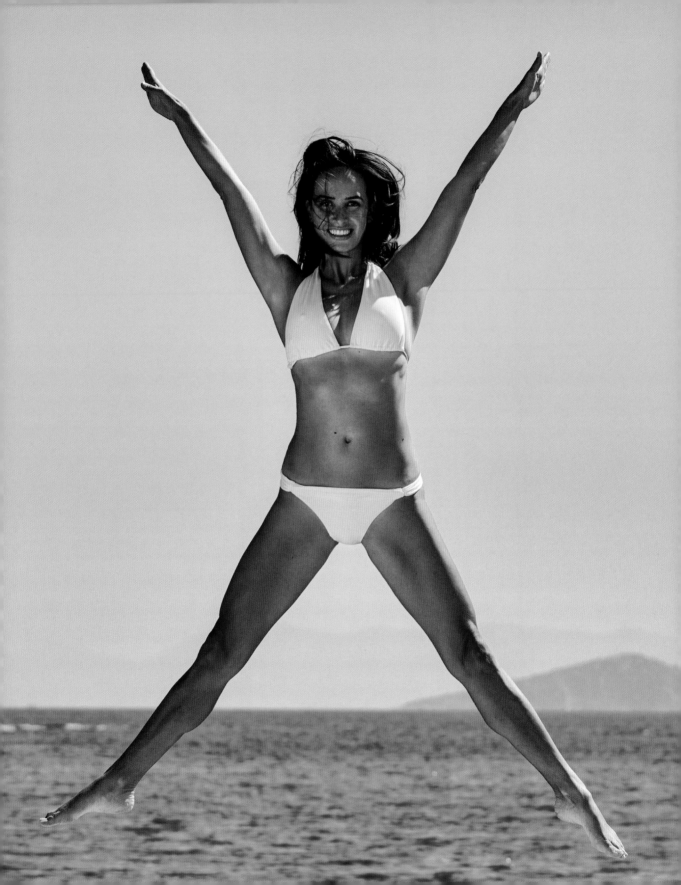

III MOVEMENT

Movement is magical.

Don't be one of those annoying people who says, "I hate exercise." You don't. You just need to find exercise you enjoy. I've lost count of the number of people I've turned from hating exercise to valuing their bodies, cherishing moving them, and feeling incredible.

I've included some Bodyism circuits in this chapter. You'll see in the Bodyism two-week plan (pages 88–91) how to create a full workout using these circuits. Always start with Prehab Circuit (pages 62–63) and end with the Regenerate Circuit (pages 72–73). Try to include two of the other circuits, repeated two or three times.

Why is movement a pillar of health?

Movement is medicine for the body and for the mind. Our bodies need to move, so we deserve to do that. Almost every day, a new published study proves the benefits of exercise. The benefits aren't just physical, they're psychological, too. In April 2014, the University of Eastern Finland found that physical activity can protect against dementia in old age. Researchers found that participants who engaged in physical activity at least twice a week had a much lower risk of dementia than those who were less active.

Movement literally will make you smarter. It directly relates to cognitive ability, a decreased risk of mental illness and degenerative diseases, and generally leads to being happier and healthier for longer. If you need any more convincing about why movement is a pillar of health, then this book isn't for you. Put it down and go eat a doughnut.

When I say "movement," I mean exercise. That doesn't mean lifting weights until your ears bleed or putting on hot pants and jumping up and down for an hour and a half every day. It can be a walk with an intelligent, gentle stretching program and a couple of body-weight resistance circuits per week. That's all you need for a long, healthy, happy life. If every day you went for a 45-minute walk, did some gentle stretching, and a few squats and lunges alongside eating and sleeping well, you'd be well on the way to being healthy, slim, and full of energy. That could be you. You don't even have to do anything crazy to get there; you just have to be kind to your body.

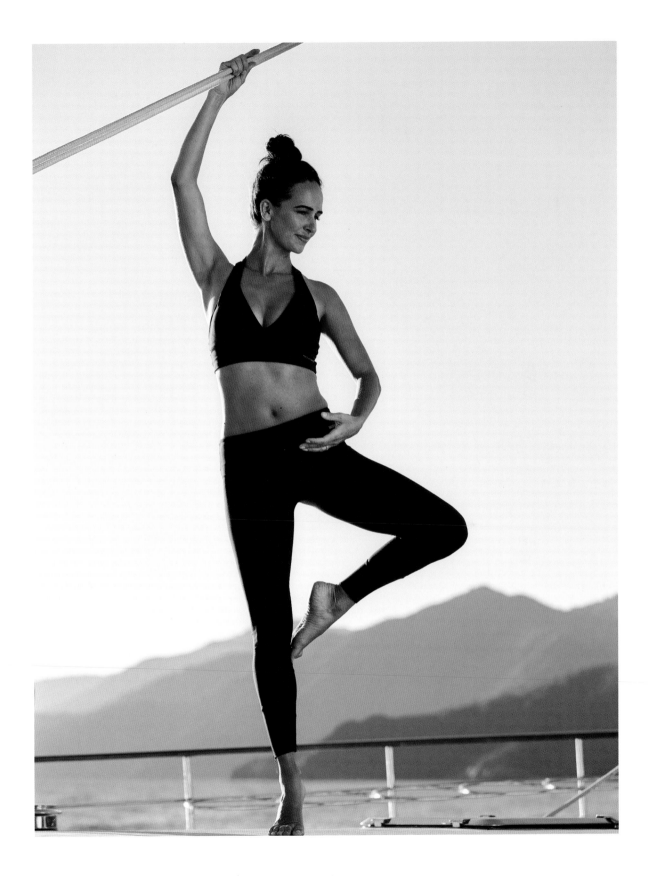

How often should I move?

Everyone always asks this question. A better question is, "How often do I have the privilege and the joy of moving?" Your body loves to move, so be grateful that you can move your body and do it every day.

Find time to move every day in different ways, and don't just stick to the gym. Carry your children, walk in the park, or offer to give someone a piggyback ride to work from the bus stop. Kidding! . . . but you get the point. Embrace change. I'm a creature of habit and really comfortable being comfortable. When I've opened my mind and tried something new, I've never regretted it (apart from that tap-dancing club . . . I still regret that).

Thinking of exercise in the same way that we think about food illustrates why balance and variety are so important. Is broccoli good for us? Yes, absolutely. Should we just eat broccoli every day and nothing else? Absolutely not. That would be stupid and unhealthy. If you did that, you'd have an eating disorder.

Ask the same question with exercise: is running good for you? Yes, it is. Is it all I need to do? Absolutely not. Just like nutrition, be balanced about it.

I'm more than 40 years old, and I've never been in better shape. I train less than ever, but I mix it up. I lift weights for 20 minutes twice a week, I do yoga, and my great joy is jiu-jitsu three times a week.

The circuits in this chapter will show you safe, effective exercises to get you started. Sign up for something new, be careful, and constantly come back to the question, "Am I being kind to myself?"

Why do I need to warm up?

What we consider "warming up" isn't what it was ten years ago. It doesn't mean 20 minutes on the treadmill; it means intelligent, targeted movement prep.

It's called movement prep because it literally prepares your body for movement. It activates the right muscles so that you achieve results in less time, prevent injury, and optimize your workout.

Hip extensions switch on your glutes (and help perk your butt), plank variations switch on your abdominals, supermans activate your postural muscles and connect your arms and legs with your abs. All of these movements have powerful reasons behind them, and they're a simple, effective way of preparing your body for whatever movement you're about to do.

Movement prep amplifies your workout and makes it safer. You need to get your body and mind ready to move if you want to enhance your performance and prevent injury.

How long should I train?

Some people want to train for 90 minutes or two hours. If you're training for that long, you're doing it wrong because you're not doing it smart enough. You can make significant progress with your body, without damaging it, by working the three aspects of movement intelligently:

1. Balance. Movements that challenge your balance include single leg work, single arm work, certain yoga poses, and even closing your eyes while doing a familiar movement, such as a squat or a lunge, or even a push-up. You'll be surprised how much more demanding that is.

2. **Strength.** This can be anything from lifting weights to bodyweight exercises, such as squats, single lunges, push-ups, or, if you're ready for it, handstands.

3. **Cardio.** This includes the full spectrum, from sustained cardio, such as a long walk in the park, to high-intensity cardio, such as sprints in the gym.

A really good, balanced program incorporates all three of these. Even if you're training for a marathon, it's important to implement all three aspects of exercise. If you run without doing joint stabilization, strength work, and skill-based balance work, you face a greater chance of injury through faulty movement patterns and unstable joints.

Just remember, as we've said many times before, life is long, so a workout should amplify your enjoyment of it rather than break your body down or become joyless and obsessive. Nourish your body.

Is running good or bad?

It's both. It's great because it's free, you can start immediately, and you can do it just about anywhere in the world. On the flip side, it often becomes obsessive, destructive, and can cause long-term damage if you overdo it. It's one of the first things Hollywood stylists and anti-aging experts tell you to stop doing because it causes facial sagging and because of the amount of oxidative stress it puts on your system. Running is great if it's your only option, but there are so many better ways of getting a healthy, happy body. If you love running, then go for it, enjoy it, but please be balanced and include strength training in your workout. If you're running in the park, always do your movement prep and find a bench on which to do some tricep dips, lunges, and squats.

Is cycling good or bad?

Cycling is a repetitive movement pattern, so it can reduce your athletic ability in terms of motor skills and coordination. Cyclists and rowers can suffer from significant back pain. I'm saying this so you know the side effects as well as the benefits. I'm *not* saying, "Avoid cycling." It's fantastic as long as it forms part of a balanced, intelligent program that nourishes and works your entire body. If it brings you joy, then great, but incorporate movement prep and make sure you add the Bodyism circuits into your week.

How long will it take me to see results?

That depends what you mean by "results." As we know, any change that happens in your body happens in your mind first. The second that you commit to being kind to yourself and living a long, happy, healthy life is the moment that you undergo the most important and powerful transformation, the change in your mind. The rest is easy. Then you'll start to see the results in your body quickly. The changes that you see in your body are a side effect of the wonderful changes in your mind. When you begin to enjoy the process and appreciate that life is a beautiful journey, as opposed to a series of destinations, not only do you stop thinking about results in terms of body-fat percentage or a number on a scale, but your body transforms at a breath-taking rate; this is when the fastest and most dramatic changes happen. The tricky thing is that you see it only when you stop looking for it.

In order to achieve life-changing results in an intelligent way, focus on the four pillars of health. So many people focus just on one pillar of health. For example, they exercise to extremes but aren't sleeping, their mindset is all wrong, and they're eating badly. It's not the fastest or most intelligent way of doing it. Instead, when you calmly see what needs to be done in all four pillars of health—which doesn't take long to do—and you work on them equally and intelligently, your body will transform so much faster. The desperately miserable person on the stationary bike or in the middle of a hard-core exercise class is doing long-term damage, working harder and taking longer than the Bodyism champion. You don't need to go all-out on a spinning bike to look and feel great—just try not to be smug about it.

Why is rest important?

I always thought resting was me being lazy, but rest is when the magic happens. Those rest days are when your body recharges, regenerates, and when it really burns fat and creates long, lean muscle. It's when everything optimizes.

Rest days can take many different forms. If three or four times a week you're training intensely, on the other days go for a nice walk or do some gentle yoga. If you can, book yourself a massage. The amount of rest you need depends on the level of exercise you're doing. I do jiu-jitsu three times a week, which is fairly high intensity, so on the other days I walk, do yoga, or play with the kids. Sunday is my day of complete rest from any kind of organized exercise. It's also when I try and have either a warm bath or a massage (if I'm really lucky).

How do I know if I'm overtraining?

Movement is medicine. As with all medicine, you can overdose on it. Exercise is wonderful for you, but when you do too much of it, you can ruin your body. It can cause injury, create hormonal imbalances, and lower your immune system. Here are the signs that you're overtraining.

1. Exhaustion. If you have a constant feeling of exhaustion, that's not good. It's great to push yourself every now and then, and feeling exhausted from your workout can feel really fulfilling. It becomes a problem when it happens four times a week and you walk out of the gym completely depleted—especially when you combine this with poor food choices. You're depleting your system and undernourishing yourself. Eventually you'll get sick and injured. This isn't an if, it's a when. It happens all the time. People burn out. It's great to train and test your limits, but do it intelligently and make sure you nourish your body with good-quality food and good-quality rest.

2. Poor food choices. People who overtrain tend to make poor food choices alongside their workouts. Either they reward themselves with processed foods or a sugar-filled treat with no protein or nutritional value—and then push themselves to work even harder in the gym the next day—or they choose foods that don't allow their bodies to recover and replenish. They might have coffee and steamed lettuce leaves, thinking that's the only way to lose weight, and their bodies will go into starvation mode right away. They might see short-term results, but that won't ever work for the long term.

3. Niggling Injuries. This is your body's powerful way of telling you that what you're doing isn't working. Don't ignore it; listen to it. That constant pain in your knee, hip, back, or wherever is your body telling you to fix something. If you train through it and you're not a professional athlete, you have a real issue. Pain is a way your body communicates with you, so find someone who can help you with that injury. Lower back pain can come from not enough exercise because your muscles are weak, or it can come from too much exercise because you're doing the wrong thing constantly. If you notice frequent aches and pains, don't ignore them. This happens a lot to spinners because people often compromise their postures on the bike, which can put unnecessary pressure on their backs.

4. **Dreading training.** If you're dreading it and it's no fun anymore, something's not working for you. Keep searching for what you love.

5. **Always prioritizing exercise above everything.** Make exercise part of your life, but don't let it get in the way of your life. Some people choose exercise over anything and everything. Don't miss out on the rest of your life in order to do an extra session at the gym. You'll regret it later. Make sure you're choosing exercise because you want to do it and it feels right. An agent in New York once told me that he was going spinning in the morning and again in the evening. He was proudly addicted. That kind of punishing schedule of hard-core, high-intensity exercise does long-term damage. Remember, your body loves to move every day, but that doesn't mean you have to go to a high-intensity class every day. Walking is just as amazing.

6. **Weight gain.** The biology of overtraining often creates a high production of cortisol, the stress hormone that dumps fat on the front of the tummy. Yes, you literally can run yourself fat. Sometimes, I work with clients who aren't eating enough and are exercising too much, which prevents them from losing weight because they're in a constant state of starvation mode. Their bodies aren't willing to let go of the fat. That's where the magic of being intelligent about the four pillars really comes into play. If you nourish yourself properly by eating more good-quality foods, your body will feel amazing and won't find itself in a constant state of fight or flight. When you go to crazy high-intensity classes all the time, you're working against your body, not with it.

Top Tip Manage your movement habit. Many people are addicted to exercise, and they're ruining their bodies because of it. Address whatever belief is driving you to do that amount of exercise. It's about managing that situation and always coming back to being kind to yourself. I'm addicted to exercise, but I manage it. If, like me, you don't feel good if you haven't exercised, that doesn't mean that you have to do spinning or high-intensity interval training every day. Change your mindset and remind yourself that any movement is great—a long walk, a swim, yoga, a dance class, boxing, lifting—and will keep you feeling brilliant. Make sure it's balanced. I've been stuck in the rut of doing the same thing every day. It's all about scheduling, so put in your diary or calendar: yoga today, weights tomorrow, etc. Once it's written down, look at it. If it's all high intensity, change it up.

If you're an exercise addict, you'll understand what I'm saying here. If you're not and this makes no sense, then don't worry. This doesn't apply to you. If it's Thursday and you haven't moved since last Friday's exercise class and you're wondering if you're overdoing it, this word of warning isn't for you. Make the changes that will help you and follow the principles of being kind to yourself.

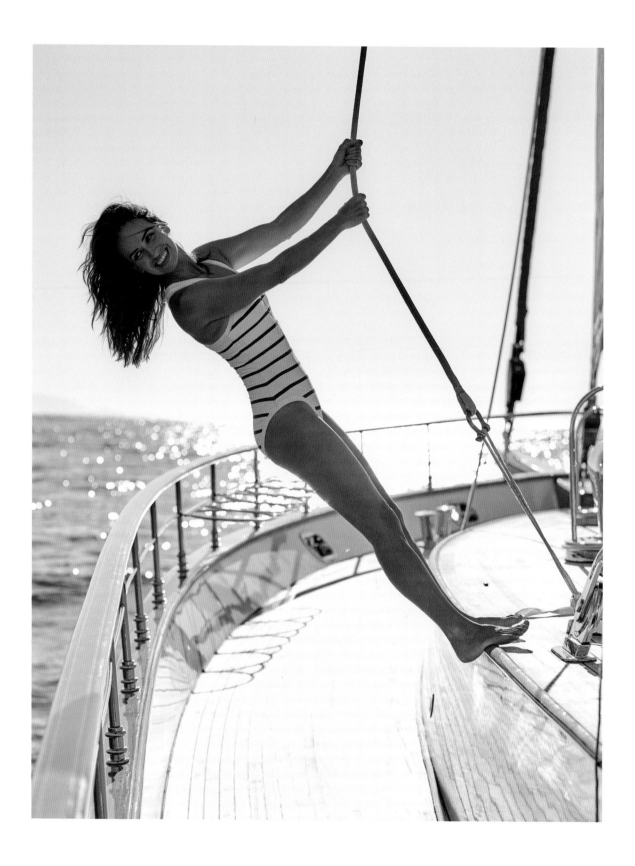

How do you get back on track after a big slip?

Living well needs to become part of your life, rather than controlling your life. You don't need to spend hours making healthy food. You don't need to train for an hour a day. (Our circuits take fewer than 20 minutes.) You just need to move your body every day and eat nourishing foods.

After Chrissy had our daughter, Charlotte, the first thing she did was walk. She didn't need to start with yoga or Pilates. Just walking and getting in touch with her body again were exactly what she needed.

Christiane Duigan: My biggest tip is to start slowly. When I began exercising again, I started off doing one or two hip extensions at a time, then I slowly built it up. Alongside this, I walked every day and did pelvic floor exercises. I kept an eye on my posture, because good posture makes you look slimmer and strengthens your core, which helps your stomach muscles fuse back together. I didn't need to lift weights because I was lifting Charlotte all the time. I didn't deprive myself, I didn't cut out any food groups, I just ate healthy foods, and I listened to my body. I took my time and I'm glad I did, because when weight comes off slowly and steadily, it stays off for longer. Remember, you don't need to rush. Be kind and respectful to yourself.

Will exercise ever feel fun?

It's all about how you approach something. When you realize that you are lucky to be able to move, it changes things. Remember, exercise doesn't mean you have to wear hot pants and dance around like a maniac for an hour. It can take the form of a long walk, squats, lunges, press-ups, and dips in your living room, or going to your local gym and connecting with other human beings. When it's not fun, change it up.

For me, surfing and jiu-jitsu are constantly inspiring, creative and fun. Of course, there are times when they're challenging, but I value those times too, because I can transcend any difficulties and then transfer that determination into my life. It creates strength and the ability to keep going when I'm uncomfortable or feel like giving up. I've learned so much from being a very bad surfer, trying to get out through big waves and never giving up. Every time I do makes me stronger and more determined. It's the same with jiu-jitsu: I don't have a natural talent, but what I've developed is a real strength of purpose and will. I won't give up; sometimes I lose (in fact, often I lose), but I never get beaten (what this means is I won't quit), and that inspires me in my daily life. Find the value in exercising and moving.

Why do I lose weight on vacation?

Because you're relaxed. That's the shortest, most correct, most complete answer. The science remains the same: when your body and mind let go and stop stressing and obsessing, that not only enables you to lose weight, but ongoing intolerances also can disappear. It's an incredible example of how what you think can affect how you feel and how you look. Take what you notice about your behavior on vacation back home with you. For example, on vacation, we always spend more time enjoying our meals. We eat slowly and calmly, which gives us our best chance to listen to our bodies. A vacation takes us away from our daily stresses, enabling us to metabolize better, digest better, and be more mindful than normal.

How do you know when to go from losing weight to maintaining a healthy weight?

What's amazing about the human body is that you don't need to worry about that. When you're nourishing yourself, moving intelligently, and being kind to yourself, your body will go to its ideal weight. As soon as you're treating it right, you won't need to restrain yourself; your body will know, and you'll feel energized and right. If you're being kind to yourself, you'll be listening to what your body wants and not feel like you're restricting yourself in any way. The moment you're in tune with your body, you won't need to think about losing weight.

Where do I start if I'm severely overweight, have joint problems and lost any motivation?

First, you're not alone. So many people are in exactly the same or a very similar situation. By following the Blueprint, so many of those issues will disappear more quickly than you can imagine. By nourishing your body and by doing some gentle movement every single day, you will notice profound changes not just in how you look but also how you feel.

Be more powerful than all of your excuses.

How can I lift my butt?

Resistance bands are one of the only pieces of equipment we use. They're incredibly effective and an intelligent way to lift your butt without overworking the quads, a common problem for people who sit at a desk every day. Exercises can include band-walking and hip extensions. The bands enable you to work your butt without damaging your knees, hips, or ankles. That helps stabilize those joints, too. Elite athletes warm up with these bands. If you don't have or want the bands, then hip extensions and squat thrusts are your butt's best friend. Another great thing to do is to squeeze your glutes whenever you can. Standing in line at the supermarket? Waiting to pick up the kids from school? Squeeze your butt for 10 seconds as hard as you can, then rest for 10 seconds. Doing this every day will give you a smoking hot butt. Just don't do it while you walk because it'll look like you urgently need a bathroom!

How do I get a flat tummy?

A flat tummy won't make you happy, but being happy will give you a flat tummy.

One of my clients always said, "I'm training until I get there." I asked, "Until you get where?" and she replied, "Until I lose weight and get abs." I said, "You'll never get there because you are always here."

Remember, you're always where you are in the present moment; it's not when, it's now and here. My client smartly and quickly realized that when doesn't exist.

All the things that make people happy—less stress, nourishing foods, a good night's sleep—will lead to a flat tummy as a by-product. Also, a flat tummy is way more than doing crunches. Your stomach is almost like a second brain. It's no accident that we call it "gut instinct" or a "gut feeling." So much of our mindset is emotionally driven. If you can find ways to relieve your stress, you'll see the effects in your tummy. Also, healing your gut solves so many seemingly unrelated problems—emotionally, physically, and hormonally. Get your digestion right, and everything else is easy (pages 24–45).

How can I make my legs long and lean?

Can you have the appearance of longer, leaner legs? Absolutely.

If the majority of your exercise consists of spinning, squats and lunges, running, and other shortening exercises, chances are your legs won't look long and lean. To achieve that long and lean aesthetic, add lengthening exercises, such as yoga, Pilates, and ballet, as well as postural exercises, which offer the quickest way of giving the appearance of weight loss. Also a small amount of cardio and lifting. Cardio includes long, sustained movement, such as walking, and also quick high-intensity cardio bursts, which raise your heart rate. Your attitude to exercise reflects in your body. If you're obsessive and only lift weights, your body will reflect that.

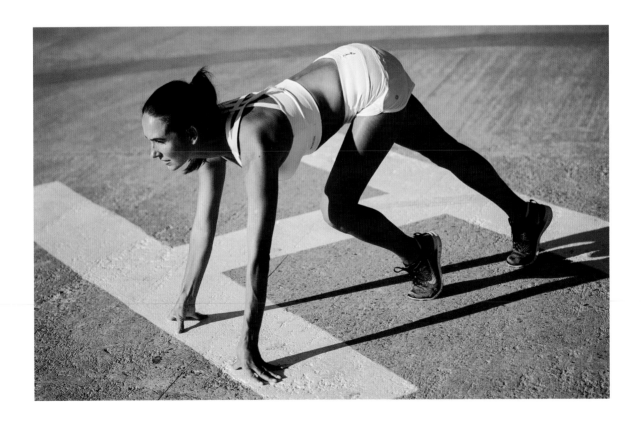

Will weightlifting make women bulky?

The science suggests not. It can't make women bulky because of their relatively low levels of testosterone and the way they are built, biochemically and mechanically. But be intelligent about it. If you don't want to look like a bodybuilder, don't train like a bodybuilder. If you're doing heavy-weighted squats, deadlifts, and lunges every day, eventually your legs will adapt. The problem is that most women are quad-dominant. They activate their quads more than their glutes and hamstrings. Because we all spend so much time sitting down, big quads give the appearance of bulky legs more than anything else. Incorporate lengthening exercises, such as yoga, Pilates, and stretching into weight sessions, and add some quick cardio bursts. That's how you get results that will reduce the likelihood of bulking up. Lifting weights won't necessarily bulk you up, but you need to learn to manage your program well. Lifting two or three times a week will keep your bones strong and healthy, help you maintain lean muscle mass, and keep your connective tissue strong. If you're lifting to the point of injury and exhaustion, pull it back. You are your own expert.

Final word on movement

Don't underestimate the importance of stretching. Give your body time to return to its normal rhythm after exercising so you can feel refreshed, mindful, and re-energized when you finish your workout. The Regenerate Circuit on pages 72–73 will help you do just that.

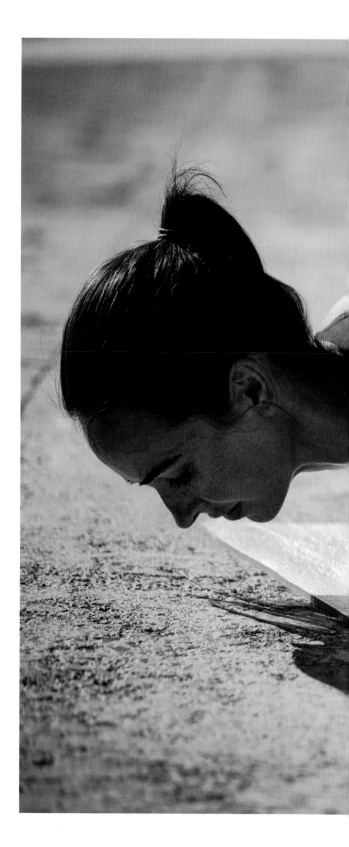

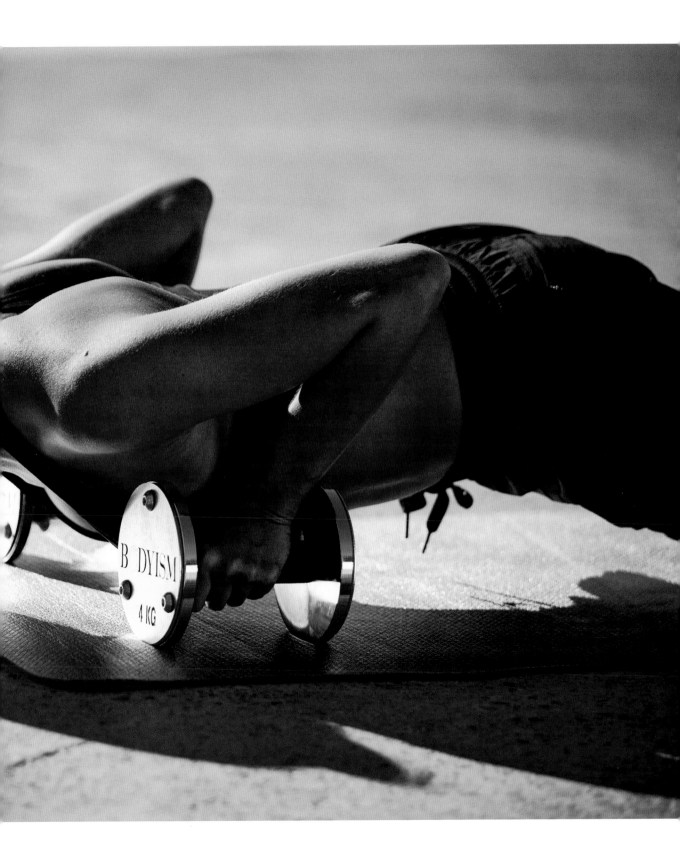

BODYISM
EXERCISES

Here are some of our best-loved exercise circuits.
As I always say, you are your own expert so choose
the exercises that you enjoy the most, mix and
match, and find the joy in moving your body. Always
remember to start with the Prehab Circuit (pages
62–63) to warm up those muscles and end with the
Regenerate Circuit (pages 72–73) to, well, regenerate.

Each time you exercise, choose two of the circuits
from the selection in the following pages (Perky Butt,
Long Lean Legs, Flat-Tummy or Perfect Posture)
and repeat the first circuit twice. Next, complete the
Quick Cardio Burst (opposite). For the second circuit,
do it twice, then follow immediately with a second
round of the Quick Cardio Burst. Finish with the
Regenerate Circuit and always remember: your body
loves to move.

Follow the at-a-glance chart below once you are in
the swing of things.

WARM UP

**1x Prehab Circuit
(pages 62–63)**

CIRCUITS

**2x circuit of your choice
(pages 64–71)**

**1x Quick Cardio Burst
(opposite)**

**2x circuit of your choice
(pages 64–71)**

**1x Quick Cardio Burst
(opposite)**

COOL DOWN

**1x Regenerate Circuit
(pages 72–73)**

QUICK CARDIO BURST

Hand Walkouts
(30 seconds)

1. Stand up straight with hands in the air.

2. Bring your hands down to the ground and walk them forward until you are in a plank position. Make sure you brace your glutes and abs and then walk your hands further forward.

3. Reverse the movement by walking your hands back to the starting position and stand with your hands in the air again. Keep your head even with your spine.

4. Repeat as fast as you can for 30 seconds.

Mountain Climbers
(30 seconds)

1. Begin in a push-up position with hands under shoulders, back flat, feet together and belly button drawn in.

2. Keep your core tight, bring one knee forward toward your chest, then straighten your leg back out behind you.

3. Repeat with the opposite leg and continue for 30 seconds as fast as you can.

Burpees, no jump
(30 seconds)

1. Stand up straight with your feet shoulder-width apart. Sink back into a squat position, with your backside pushed out as if to sit down. Sink further to go from a squat to a crouch.

2. Put your hands on the floor in front of you, shoulder-width apart.

3. Hop back with your feet, into a plank position. Make your body a straight line from your head to your ankles. Line up your shoulders with your wrists. Keep your body straight—don't arch your backside up or droop at the waist.

4. Bring your feet back to your hands with a quick hop.

5. Stand up to return to the starting position. Repeat as fast as you can, for 30 seconds.

Alternating Disco Lunge
(30 seconds)

1. Begin standing in an upright position with feet together and perfect posture (stand up straight, keep your back straight, with your ears over your shoulders and your shoulders over your hips. Look straight ahead and think tall, right through your spine and through the top of your head). Begin with your arms by your sides, with hands clenched, thumbs up.

2. Set your core by drawing in your belly button and step forward into a lunge.

3. As you lunge forward with your left foot, extend both arms above your head to make a Y shape. Land heel then toe and let your front knee bend forward.

4. Push back to the starting position with your arms by your sides. Repeat for 30 seconds.

Top Tip Repeat each exercise for 30 seconds and then rest for 15 seconds. Repeat the whole circuit four times. It's an awesome cardio burst.

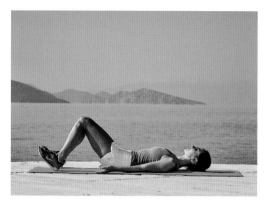
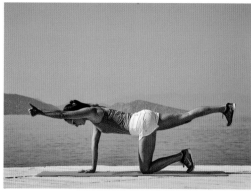
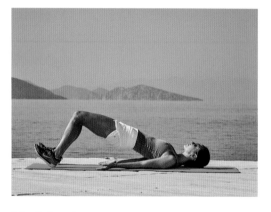
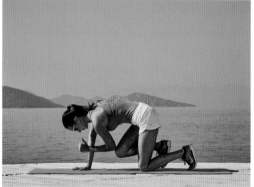

Hip Extension
(10–12 repetitions)

1. Lie on your back with your knees bent.

2. Exhale and roll your pelvis to lift your glutes and lower back off the ground. Try to create a straight line from your shoulders to your knees.

3. Pause at the top while squeezing your glutes, then reverse the movement, rolling each vertebra of the spine back to the starting position. Remember to use your glutes in this movement rather than over-working your lower back. Repeat 10–12 times.

Top Tip Every time you do one of these circuits, make sure you hold your stomach in and really activate your glutes (clench your butt)!

Supermans
(10–12 repetitions, both sides)

1. Begin on your hands and knees with toes firmly pointed into the floor. Make sure your spine and neck are in a neutral position, with hands under shoulders and knees under hips.

2. Extend your right arm out in front of you alongside your head, thumb up, while you extend your left leg backward, toes still pointing down. Imagine you are being pulled from either end.

3. Bring your arm and leg in underneath your torso simultaneously so they touch. Repeat 10–12 times before switching sides.

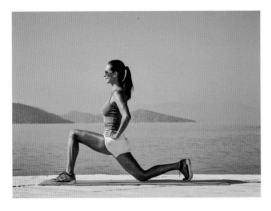

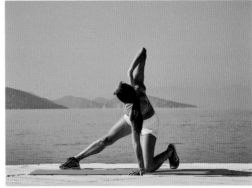

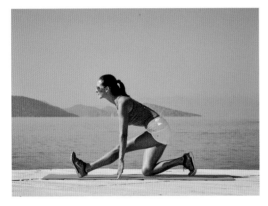

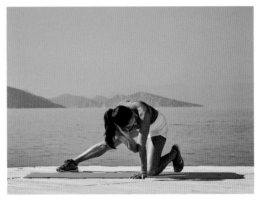

Hip to Hamstring
(10 repetitions, both sides)

1. Place your left foot flat on the ground and your right knee on a soft pad or mat on the ground.

2. Rest your left hand on the knee of your front leg.

3. Lean slightly forward with your torso, tighten your stomach, and contract the glute of your back leg.

4. Maintaining this position, shift your entire body slightly forward. Then move your hips backward, straightening your front leg and moving forward with your torso to stretch the hamstring. Repeat 10 times before switching sides.

Thoracic Rotation with Adductor Stretch
(10 repetitions, both sides)

1. Start on all fours with your hands under your shoulders, one knee under your hip, the other straight out to the side with the foot against the floor.

2. With the hand on the same side as the outstretched leg, salute to your head, and rotate your torso through your shoulder blades so the elbow of your saluting arm points toward the ceiling or sky.

3. Return back slowly, touch elbow to elbow, then return to the start position. Repeat 10 times before switching sides.

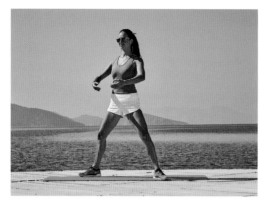

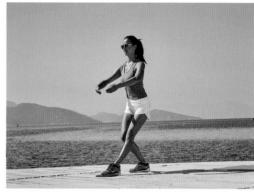

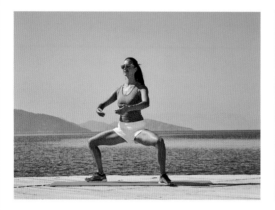

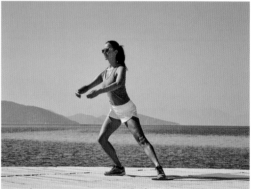

Goddess to Relieve Squat
(12–15 repetitions)

1. Stand with your arms straight out in front at shoulder height, feet wider than shoulder-width apart and toes pointed out at 45 degrees. Keep your core engaged by drawing your belly button in toward your spine.

2. Initiate the movement by pushing the hips back and bending the knees so you squat back and down until your thighs are parallel to the floor. Return to the standing position by pushing through the hips and the heels while keeping your torso upright. Repeat 12–15 times.

Rainbow Slide with Gliders
(12–15 repetitions, both sides)

1. Stand with your arms out in front of you, feet shoulder-width apart with your toes on a Bodyism gliding disc on each side. If you don't have the discs, use a small paper plate—it works in a similar way!

2. Slide your left foot in front of you and then arc it out to the left, holding on to the disc as you go. Keep your right knee bent throughout.

3. Reverse the movement, returning briefly to the starting position while keeping your right knee bent. Repeat the sequence 12–15 times before repeating on the other foot.

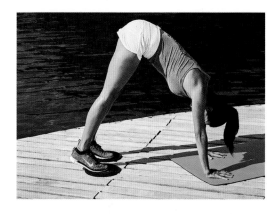

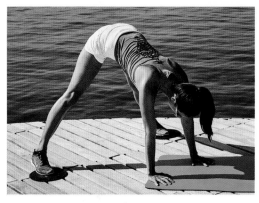

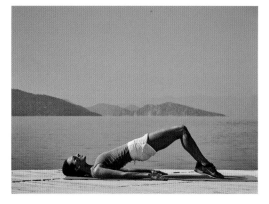

Pike Adductor
(12–15 repetitions)

1. Step onto two Bodyism gliding discs or small paper plates and start in a pike position. With arms and legs straight, plant your hands directly under your shoulders to make your butt the highest point. Keep the weight in your hands and toes and relax your shoulders.

2. Tighten your core and glutes and drive your legs to a wide stance, taking the discs with you as you go. Reverse the movement back to the starting position. Repeat 12–15 times.

Hip Extension on Toes
(15 repetitions)

1. Lie on your back with both knees bent, toes on the ground and heels in the air.

2. Lift your hips off the ground, raising them as high as you can go, squeezing your glutes together and keeping your core tight.

3. Pause at the top for 1 second, then return to the start position. Repeat 15 times.

PERKY BUTT CIRCUIT

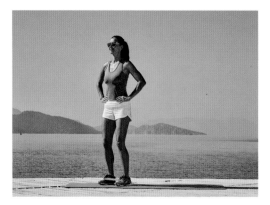

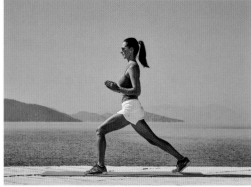

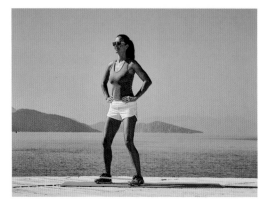

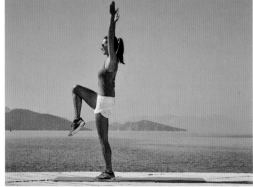

**Tube Walking
(3 repetitions)**

1. Stand in a quarter-squat position, with your feet hip-width apart and place a Bodyism mini band around your feet making sure it is taut. If you don't have a Bodyism band, you can use another exercise band.

2. Walk to the side with small steps for 10 strides and then walk back, leading with the opposite leg. Repeat three times.

**Rocket Lunge
(10 repetitions, both sides)**

1. Take a step back with your left foot, bending both knees at 90 degrees, so your back knee hovers off the floor.

2. Extend both knees and transfer your weight on to your right foot. At the same time, lift up your left foot, bringing your knee to your chest while raising your arms to the ceiling.

3. Release your left leg from your chest and place it back on the floor in the starting lunge position. Repeat 10 times on each side.

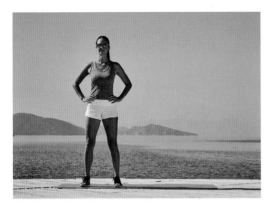

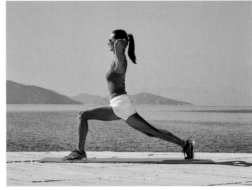

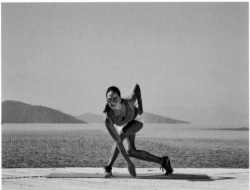

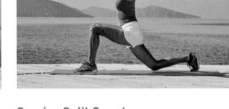

Drop Step Lunge with Reach
(10 repetitions, both sides)

1. From a standing position with hands on hips, take a big step back with your right foot and move it behind the left foot. Once your right foot makes contact with the ground, square your hips, chest, and feet so they all are facing forward.

2. Sit back slowly and drop your back knee toward the ground while reaching across your torso with your right hand. Feel the stretch in the outside of your thigh and your glutes. Keep your chest up and body squared, facing forward, the entire time.

3. Stand back up to return to the starting position. Repeat 10 times, then reset on the opposite side.

Sunrise Split Squat
(10 repetitions, both sides)

1. Stand in a staggered stance, with right foot in front of left, with your hands on your head.

2. Begin by lowering yourself down (not forward) until your left knee is almost touching the ground. Pause, then push yourself back up to starting position. Repeat 10 times with your right foot forward and then repeat with the left foot forward.

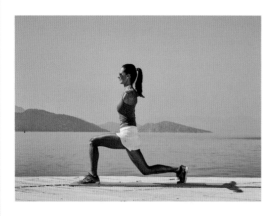

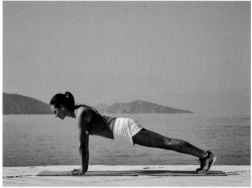

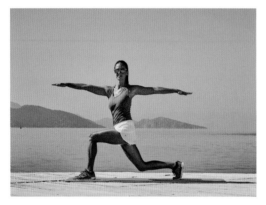

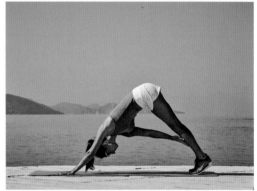

FLAT-TUMMY CIRCUIT

Lunge Twist
(10 repetitions, both sides)

1. Lunge forward; keep your hips facing forward, with your head still, arms out to the side parallel with the ground.

2. As you move down into the lunge, slowly rotate your torso over the lead leg, with your hands still out to the side. Keep your body upright, with your chest out and shoulders rolled back.

3. Rotate back to the middle and then return to the starting position. Repeat 10 times, then continue with the other leg.

High Plank to Shin Tap
(10 repetitions, both sides)

1. Start in high-plank position, just like traditional plank but with straight arms instead of bent at the forearm.

2. Lift your right hand off the floor and reach under your torso toward your left ankle, gently tapping the front of your foot or ankle if possible.

3. Return the right hand to the floor and repeat with the opposite arm. Repeat 10 times on each side.

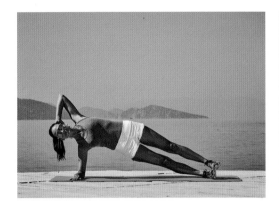

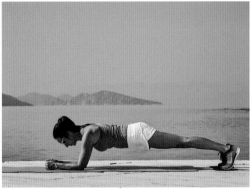

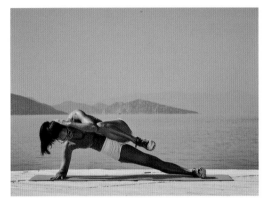

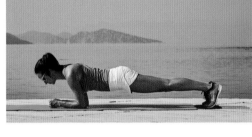

**Side Plank—Knee to Elbow
(10 repetitions, both sides)**

1. Come into a forearm side plank on your left side, with your left elbow resting on the floor below your shoulder.

2. Place your right arm behind your head and lift your right knee up toward your bent arm. Don't let your hips drop. Repeat 10 times on each side.

**The Body Saw with Gliding Discs
(10 repetitions)**

1. Start on the floor and come into a forearm plank, with your fists clenched or your palms facing up.

2. Place each foot on a Bodyism gliding disc. If you don't have the discs, use a small paper plate.

3. Keeping your body in a straight line, press your forearms into the floor (forearms should not move) to push your body backward, so your arms form a 60-degree angle.

4. Reverse the motion by pressing into your forearms to pull your body forward, back to the start position. Repeat 10 times.

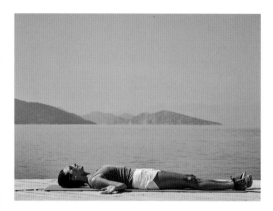

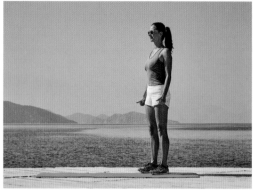

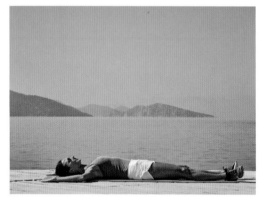

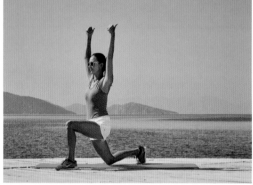

**Floor Slide
(10 repetitions)**

1. Lie on your back with your legs flat and heels on the ground. (If you find this exercise difficult, begin with your knees bent and feet on the ground.)

2. Place both arms out at shoulder height on the floor, with elbows bent at 90 degrees.

3. Tuck in your chin, engage your torso, and slowly slide both arms up along the floor toward your head, without letting your lower back, rib cage, shoulders, or chin lift.

4. Stop at the top and slide your arms back to the starting position. Repeat 10 times.

**Disco Lunge
(10 repetitions, both sides)**

1. Start with your feet hip-width apart, hands by your sides and thumbs up.

2. Step forward with your left leg and bend your knee to 90 degrees. Let your back leg follow that movement.

3. As you sink into your lunge, let your arms swing upward, beside your ears.

4. As you step back to the starting position, let your arms return to neutral. Repeat 10 times on each leg.

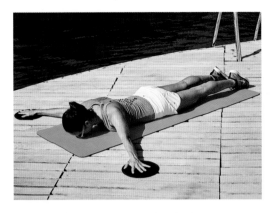

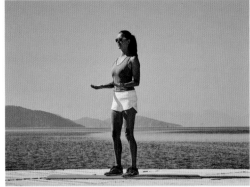

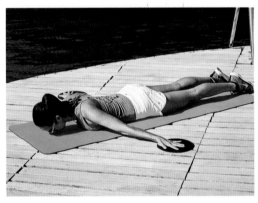

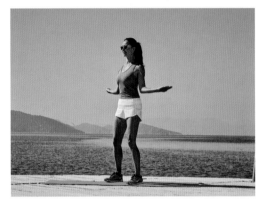

**Prone Slider Opener
(10 repetitions)**

1. Lie face down on the floor with your arms out to the sides, in line with your shoulders, and both palms facing down, resting on Bodyism gliding discs or paper plates.

2. Initiate the movement by squeezing your shoulder blades together and slightly raising your upper chest a few inches off the floor while simultaneously lowering your arms toward your sides.

3. Hold and squeeze before returning to the starting position. Repeat 10 times.

**Begging-Man Pose
(10 repetitions)**

1. Begin with feet hip-width apart, elbows bent at 90 degrees and squeezing gently at the sides of your ribcage. Place your forearms forward, with palms up and hands open. Inhale into your mid-back, pressing your shoulder blades down.

2. On the exhale, move your forearms out to the sides, keeping your elbows tucked in close to your ribs.

3. On the inhale, bring your forearms forward again, keeping your hands in front of your elbows. Feel the bottom tips of your shoulder blades squeezing toward your spine. Repeat 10 times.

REGENERATE CIRCUIT

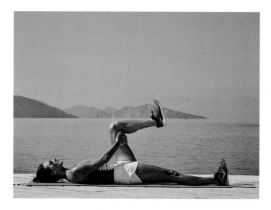

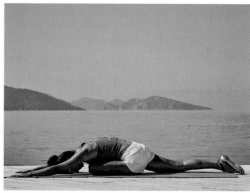

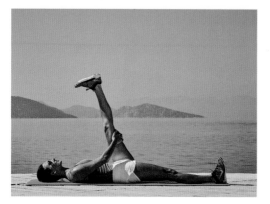

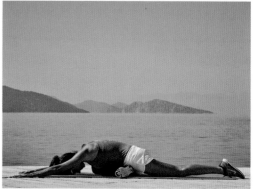

Active Leg Raise
(10 repetitions, both sides)

1. Lie on your back, with both legs straight.

2. Pull one knee toward your chest, grasping behind the knee with both hands. Straighten your lower leg as much as possible, without letting your knee move away from your chest.

3. Hold the stretch for two seconds. Relax and return to the starting position. Complete 10 repetitions on one side before repeating with the opposite leg.

Pigeon Stretch
(30 seconds, both sides)

1. Slide your right knee forward, toward your right hand, keeping your foot facing toes-down on the floor.

2 Angle your right knee at two o'clock. Slide your left leg back as far as your hips will allow.

3. Keep your hips square to the floor.

4. Keeping your torso upright, reach down to steady yourself with your hands on the floor. Try to sink your hips forward and down. If you feel comfortable, you can fold forward with your torso to meet your right knee.

5. Hold for 30 seconds and return to the top. Then repeat on the other leg.

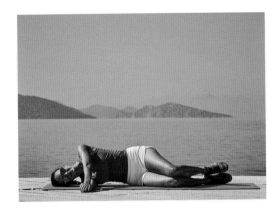

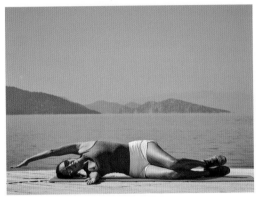

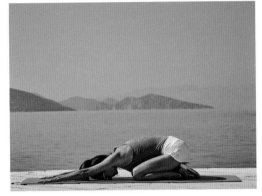

**Hug the World
(10 repetitions, both sides)**

1. Lie face up with knees bent at 90 degrees. Roll onto your right side and squeeze your thighs together, arms out in front.

2. Keeping your bottom arm and your knees pinned to the ground, rotate your chest and top arm away, trying to place your back on the ground.

3. Extend the same arm and sweep it along the ground toward your head, until it is straight overhead, then sweep it down again behind you, toward your butt and back over to the starting position. Repeat 10 times on one side before switching legs and repeating with the opposite arm.

**Child's Pose
(1–2 minutes)**

1. Get on your hands and knees and walk your hands away, in front of you.

2. Lower your buttocks down to sit on your heels. Let your arms drag along the floor as you sit back, stretching your entire spine.

3. Once you settle onto your heels, bring your hands next to your feet and relax.

4. Breathe into your back. Rest your forehead on the floor. Hold this for a minute or two, until you feel recharged and ready to get on with the rest of your day.

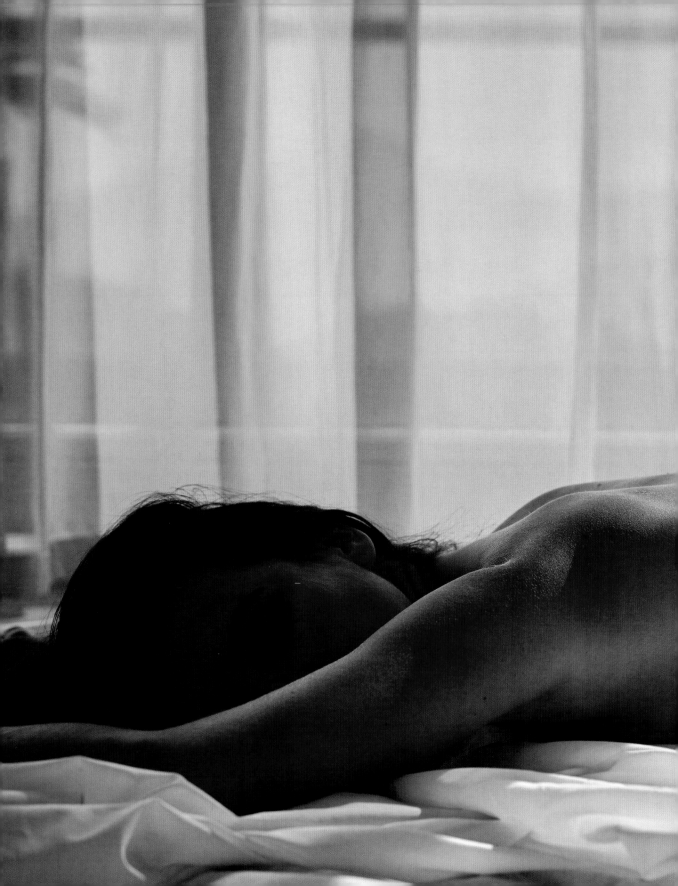

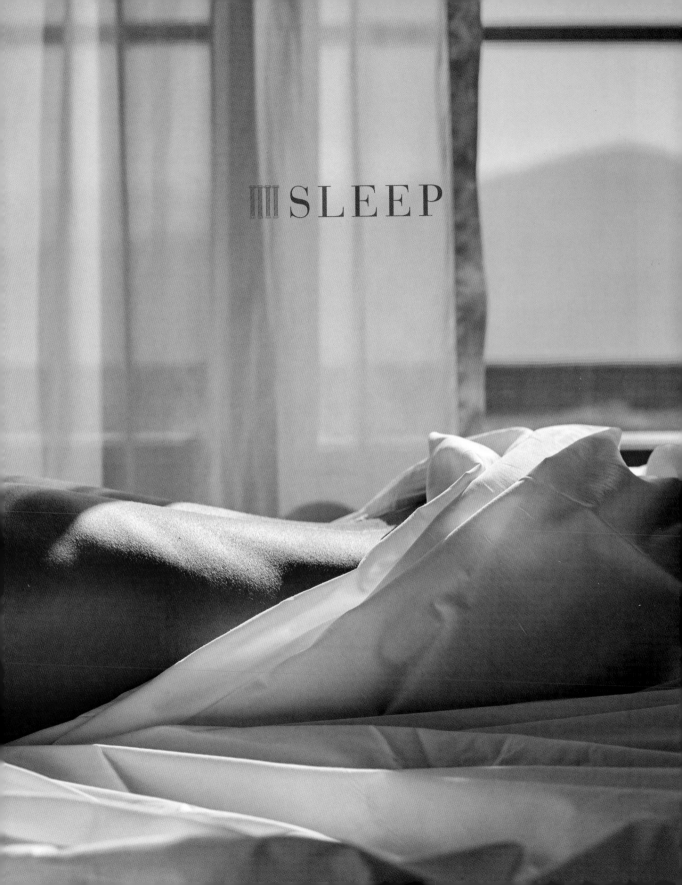

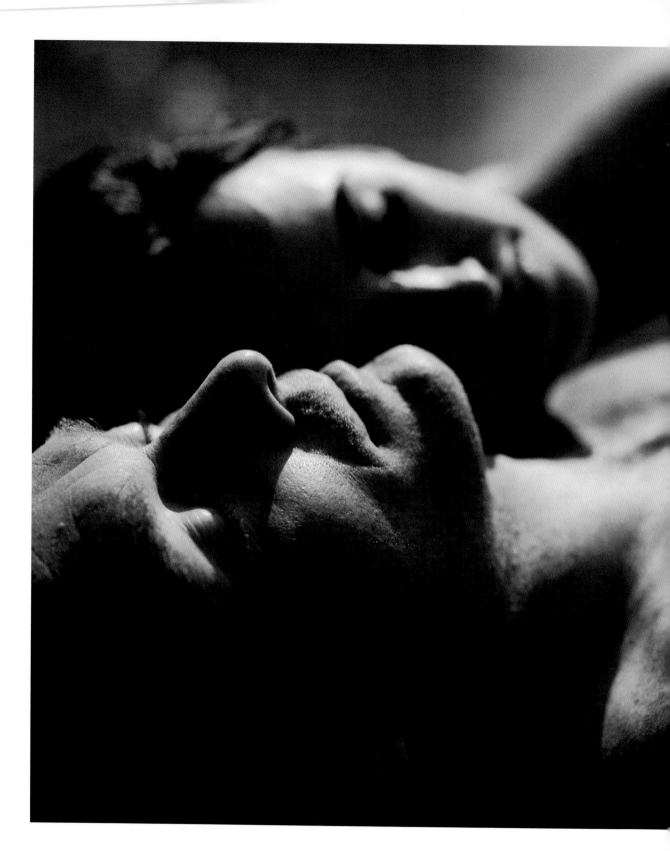

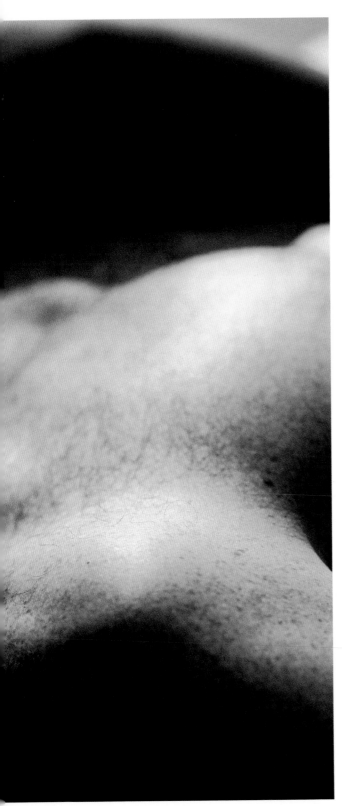

Sleep is medicine.

Why is sleep a pillar of health?

Sleep is when the magic happens. It's your body's opportunity to regenerate, recharge, and replenish. It's when everything you did throughout the day gets processed—physically, mentally, and emotionally. Without proper, good-quality sleep, any transformation to your overall wellbeing becomes difficult or close to impossible. On the wonderful flip side of that, a good night of deep, nourishing, quality sleep has the power to transform your mind and body.

If you're exercising intelligently and eating nourishing foods but not sleeping well, it's like having lots of fuel in your car but a flat tire. If I don't sleep well for a few nights in a row, I spend the day slightly hysterical and things don't feel quite right. I lose my sense of certainty and stability.

A good night's sleep will help you deal with the endless stream of Instagram bikini and butt pictures that make you want to punch your phone. It also will give your brain a much-needed chance to process all the other things going on in your life so that you wake up the next day feeling fresh, recharged, and restored.

Sleep is also the time when our body does most of its physical restoration as well as when we actually burn fat and metabolize all of the things that need to be dealt with. What I am trying to say is this: don't underestimate the importance of sleep! It is the foundation on which your health, both physical and mental, is built. Plus, when you're getting enough, it stops you acting like a crazy person.

The Biology of Sleep: When we sleep, our body gets to work; it's when the magic happens. Sleep enables the following changes to occur:

• Brain development
• Metabolism of fat
• Appetite regulation
• Immune strength improvement
• Increased creativity
• Memory enhancement

A 2014 study from Duke NUS Graduate Medical School found that the less we sleep, the faster our brains age. This obviously has a direct effect on our overall wellbeing. Another study, from Uppsala University in Sweden, showed that men who reported suffering sleep problems were one and a half times more likely to develop Alzheimer's. (Movement is another powerful way of preventing this; see pages 46–73).

Sleep is closely connected with mental health. Researchers in France have found that consistently early bedtimes help to reduce our risk of mental illness. That's because sleep disturbances affect our dopamine levels—a neurotransmitter associated with the "pleasure" part of our brains—so limited sleep can trigger depression, schizophrenia, and bipolar disorder.

Traditional Chinese medicine believes that each organ has its point of highest and lowest energy. This 24-hour cycle is thought to help us know which organs and energy channels are recharging at certain times of the night. It shows us just how vital sleep is for our body to repair optimally.

Many people make the mistake of underestimating the importance of sleep, treating it as the least essential of the four pillars. But sleep is the missing piece in the puzzle of perfect health.

Is sleep the most important pillar of all?

From the moment you wake up, if you've had a good night's sleep, you'll be more inclined to make better, kinder, and more powerful food choices and be in a better place to make decisions and react to situations in general. You'll be calmer, more centered and self-aware and less prone to ridiculous behaviour, such as tantrums, angry outbursts, and regrettable fashion statements. So, is sleep the most important pillar? It's difficult to say because, if you don't move well and eat properly, you will, in turn, have a tough time sleeping. But, on the other hand, if you don't sleep well, then you won't move with as much energy and focus, your food choices will be poorer, and your tired mental state will make life generally more difficult to deal with. If you can master getting a nourishing night's sleep, you'll find you feel less stressed and are more likely to be kind to yourself, both of which will feed into the way you approach the other three pillars.

What if I only need a few hours sleep?

Some people supposedly function brilliantly on five hours a night. I've read stories of people such as Leonardo da Vinci, Thomas Edison (who apparently developed diabetes), and other geniuses who barely slept. But, of course, aside from their famous achievements, I do wonder how happy they truly were in their day-to-day lives. (I'm not criticizing either of these people; I'm just saying that maybe we shouldn't use them as an example of how to live a happy, healthy life. . . . They obviously didn't have the time or energy for Pilates!)

In the past, I've been addicted to not sleeping. (Yes, that is a thing.) I went through a stage of going to bed at 2 a.m. and waking up for work at 5 a.m. My closest friend started to notice my mental state and worried about me. I'd wake up in the morning almost hysterical, promising myself I'd have an early night that evening, but then the evening would come round and I'd be keeping myself busy until the early hours of the morning again. I eventually collapsed into bed, completely exhausted.

The cycle went on and on. Only once I realized that it had turned into an unhealthy habit did I decide to change it.

Once I realized how important sleep was, I set out to change my relationship with it and began go to bed at the same time (10 p.m.) as often as I could and to wake up at the same time every morning. Within just two weeks, my unhealthy habit of staying up past bedtime had been replaced with a much healthier one.

Scientifically speaking, I had messed up my sleep pattern, better known as my circadian rhythm. In human beings, the circadian rhythm is determined by a small group of brain cells located in the hypothalamus (above the optic nerve). In order for our circadian rhythm to work properly, it needs constant input in the form of natural light. For example, when the light shines through the curtains in the morning, our body gears up, and when the sun sets in the evening, it will wind down, preparing us for sleep. However, modern technology has elbowed its unnaturally bright way in and messed up our natural clock, resulting in many of us having tuned out of our own circadian rhythm and making us think that we need only a few hours' sleep, when in reality we need much more.

A study by Exeter University found that "sleep almost doubles our chances of remembering previously unrecalled material." If you want to be sharp and focused in the day, you need to sleep properly the night before.

It's not just for our mental health, either, according to Dr. David Gozal, chairman of pediatrics at the University of Chicago Comer Children's Hospital. He explains that "fragmented sleep changes how the immune system deals with cancer in ways that make the disease more aggressive." Our immune system is certain to suffer if we haven't had enough rest. Dr. Axel Steiger at Munich's Max Planck Institute of Psychiatry says, "with an infection, patients become sleepy, and . . . sleep helps them recover." This is nature's way of trying to help us heal. But it only works if we let it.

What should I do to get a good night's sleep?

1. Make sleep a priority. By understanding and recognizing how important sleep is, you will start to take it more seriously.

2. It's all about creating a routine, a familiar ritual that your body and brain recognize, so you can start to unwind and prepare for a wonderful night's rest. If you can create this ritual and stick to it, you will very soon be sleeping like a baby—and I don't mean wetting the bed and crying all night! I mean the perfect peace of baby sleep, with an angelic smile across your face.

3. Try the Bodyism Serenity supplement. I spent years craving something sweet just before bed, so I spent a really long time developing this supplement so that it wouldn't raise my sugar and energy levels but would help me wind down for a great night's sleep. Serenity is my desert-island item; it's made with calming herbs that help lower anxiety levels and combat the stress hormones that dump fat on your tummy. Serenity also contains hops, oats, and camomile to help your body relax and promotes a deep, restful, rejuvenating sleep. If you can't buy it, get in the habit of having a cup of camomile tea before bed. If you really want something sweet, go for a square of bittersweet chocolate.

4. Get into bed by 10 p.m. for a 6 a.m. wake up. Eight hours is the perfect amount of sleep your body needs to achieve all the physical and mental restoration necessary during the night.

5. It may sound strange, but try to live by what I like to call the caveman approach. When the sun goes down in the evening, dim the lights in your house or apartment. Just as a caveman would light a fire at night, this is the modern-day equivalent. Limit the use of electronic devices in the evenings, such as cell phones, tablets, laptops, computers, and televisions. This further reduces external stresses on your mind and body, calming you down before

bedtime, rather than stimulating you more. It might sound silly, but it does work.

If you can apply a few of these suggestions, within just a few weeks I guarantee you will feel more energetic and less anxious. Believe it or not, the decrease in stress can also lead to a flatter tummy, too!

What if I get stressed about the fact I can't sleep?

While we need to understand the importance of sleep, we don't want that, in itself, to become a stressful factor. So many people have trouble with sleep and then spend hours worrying about it, which only creates more stress and just adds to the problem. Remind yourself that some of the most well-known meditation practitioners, such as the Dalai Lama, purposefully wake up in the middle of the night to do two to three hours of meditation. Knowing that some of the most mindful people on the planet are up in the middle of the night helps calm me down when I'm lying there, wide awake. Think of this as time when you aren't expected to do anything, and treat it as a wonderful opportunity to meditate.

What if my to-do list is keeping me awake?

I call this "spinning," when your mind is running through your endless to-do list and going round in circles. It's when you can't stop thinking of all the things you didn't get done that day and are stressing about all the things you need to do tomorrow. Spinning makes it impossible to calm your mind down and switch off. What you need to do is this: write it down, and I don't mean on your phone. Get a pen and a notebook, and write it all down. Promise yourself you will tick these things off tomorrow, then close your notebook and go to sleep or do your meditation.

Top Tip | I learned a great technique from my mother, which is a really simple meditation practice and can help relieve the pressure of feeling like you must go to sleep.

1. Close your eyes.
2. Focus on your breathing. Breathe into your stomach and feel it rise and fall.
3. Let your thoughts float in, and then out again.

This simple process is incredibly nourishing and way more beneficial than getting up and watching television, reading a book or answering emails. Eventually, you will drift off without even realizing it. Simply reframing the fact you are awake as an opportunity for you to meditate without deadlines or distractions, rather than a problem, will help calm you down, enable you to enjoy meditating, and inevitably drift off to sleep. Even if you are up all night doing it, that's fine! It's way more restful than anything else you could be doing.

Can we eat our way to better sleep?

Not necessarily, but we definitely can eat and drink our way to a bad night's sleep or, indeed, a lifetime of bad nights. Here are the main offenders:

Coffee. Relying on caffeine and sugar to get through the day can cause you to end up in a constant tired-and-wired state. I love coffee, but caffeine has a powerful effect on our bodies for much longer than we think. A study from Wayne State University and Henry Ford Hospital in Detroit, Michigan, found that consuming caffeine six hours before bed can shorten sleep by as much as one hour, so our caffeine cut-off should start well before the evening.

Late-night snacks. If you eat just before bed, your body has to work hard to digest the food while you are trying to fall asleep, which can negatively affect your circadian rhythm and therefore your sleep-wake cycle. Acid reflux is also a hugely common problem. Life sometimes get in the way, so if you do have to eat late, then choose foods that contain nutrients known to promote good sleep. Foods rich in tryptophan, such as oats, beans, rice, or turkey, are a good choice, as are foods that contain magnesium, such as seeds, nuts, leafy greens, and bananas, because magnesium can help relax your nervous system. I try not to eat anything for at least two hours before bed and drink a cup of Bodyism Serenity supplement mixed with rice milk instead—it tastes like chocolate milk!

Alcohol. Many people believe that a drink before bed helps them sleep. Alcohol is discussed in more depth in the Nutrition chapter (pages 33–35), so I will just mention here why alcohol does not help you sleep. A study carried out in 2015 by the University of Melbourne proved that alcohol works as a sleep disrupter. "The quality of sleep you get is significantly altered and disrupted," says the author of that study, Christian Nichols.

We recommended that a client who had just returned to London from New York after 10 years try the Bodyism Serenity supplement, so she swapped her nightly glass of red wine for a scoop of Serenity mixed with nut milk. She came back two weeks later and told me she'd had her best night's sleep in 10 years. She'd even got her husband, who normally made a point of not being healthy, to try it. About 30 minutes after drinking it, he took himself off to bed, whereas usually he'd have been double-screening, on his phone and the TV, until 1 a.m. It was the first time they'd felt well-rested in years!

Do I burn fat when I sleep?

Sleep deprivation results in higher levels of stress and puts our bodies on high alert for danger. This stressed-out state leads to the release of cortisol,

which in genuinely stressful situations can save your life. However, when cortisol is constantly being released, it encourages your body to store fat around your stomach. That's why so many stressed-out and sleep-deprived people hold fat on their tummies.

A 2012 Harvard Medical School study found that healthy adults who normally slept an average of 8 hours and were asked to sleep an average of 5.6 hours a night for three weeks had a decreased resting metabolic rate and increased glucose levels after meals, compared to before the experiment. Both of these effects increased their risk of obesity and diabetes.

If we haven't had a good night's sleep, the next day we're much more likely to eat foods that don't work for us. In a University of Pennsylvania study, one group of participants was kept awake all night, while another group was allowed to sleep. The people who stayed up all night ate nearly 1,000 additional calories overnight, and the next day they ate far more than the group who had slept. We know we are less decisive on little sleep (at least, I think we are . . . or maybe we're not. Oh no, I didn't sleep well last night!), so it's easy to see why we'd choose unhealthy foods and have less self-control if we haven't had a good night's sleep. Our willpower weakens, which leads to unhealthy choices.

How can I create a routine to help me sleep?

There is no single piece of advice I can give you to help you wind down for a good night's sleep, but making good habits, which help your body and mind relax before bed, will give you every chance of getting a proper rest.

One thing I've learned from my kids is that routines and rituals really help. We had to teach them how to sleep because they would lie there and didn't know how to drift off. With my daughter, Charlotte, I literally had to close her eyes for her and then I'd stay there with her until she nodded off. Charlotte and Leo have a bedtime routine which starts way before bedtime.

Their winding-down time includes a bath, a story we read from a book and a "nisery" (what Charlotte calls my made-up stories), and then we put them into bed and they go to sleep. Rituals like this are just as useful for us as adults; we just need to find our own individual winding-down routine to get our minds and bodies ready for sleep.

So how should we do it? I start winding down once I've put the kids to bed. Chrissy and I will eat dinner together, then we'll usually do another hour of work before catching up on an episode of a favorite show. We'll then switch off the TV, go to the bedroom, and we always put our phones in another room (more on this below). Then, finally, I'll have a cup of Serenity, get into bed, and, as I go to sleep, I focus on what I'm grateful for.

Despite this, I have to confess that late nights are still my vice. Every few weeks I'll still have a night where Chrissy goes to bed, but I just stay up, scrolling through my phone and watching TV, and it won't be until I'm completely exhausted that I make myself go to bed. I always feel terrible the next day. So, even while writing about the importance of this pillar, the truth is I'm still struggling to get to grips with it myself.

Why should I write a gratitude journal?

Chrissy and I have made writing a gratitude list an important part of our bedtime routine. Focusing on gratitude and being in a state of gratitude is one of the most powerful states of being. That you are grateful means something great has happened. So, finding time to be grateful is one of the best things you can do for your entire wellbeing. Think about how you feel when you are genuinely grateful. Now imagine feeling that way every minute of every day. Of course, in reality, we can't stay entirely grateful all day long, but if we can actively think of something we're genuinely grateful for, it can really help unwind the stress that has built up during the day.

For most people, it won't be, "I am grateful for the sunshine," or, "I am grateful for the cool breeze," (though great, if it is). For most people, it's more likely to be something like finding a bathroom when you really needed to pee (I can say that because we're friends now—and there are very few things that make you feel as intensely grateful as this!) or having a glass of water when you were really thirsty.

My gratitude journal focuses my mind on the blessings in my life, rather than on the list of things that might stress me out. Arianna Huffington wrote about this perfectly in her book, *The Sleep Revolution*. She explains, "it's the stresses and setbacks that seem to take center stage in our minds once our head hits the pillow. They are the preening, attention-seeking, spotlight-hogging divas of our bedtime hours, ignoring the stage manager begging them to exit. A gratitude list is a great way to knock them down a peg, shift the spotlight and make sure our blessings get the closing scene of the night."

Focus on that feeling of gratitude and try to let it consume you before you go to bed. Reserve five minutes every night for thinking about what you are truly grateful for. You can write it down (I love The Five-Minute Journal by Intelligent Change, which you can buy online worldwide), say it out loud, or simply say it in your head. I encourage you to express yourself fully and feel fine about doing so. There is nothing to be afraid of or embarrassed about. Let yourself go. What you're grateful for will change every day. Be curious and find gratitude in even the smallest of things.

Here are some things on my gratitude list:

I am grateful for my healthy body.
I am grateful for the food that I ate today.
I am grateful for the hugs that I got from my children and wife.
I am grateful that I have a home—a warm place to live in.

What's the most powerful way to start the day?

Those first few moments at the start of each day are your most powerful. Think of what you can do today to elevate it beyond yesterday. Who can you be?

Before you get up and start your day, remind yourself how powerful you are. You can do this by finding a mantra, which you can say out loud, write down or say in your head. It should be something that reminds you that you have the courage, kindness, intelligence, power, and strength to change everything.

Find words that function as your driving force, that give you your power and purpose, and that define who you are. Find words that inspire you and leave no room for pettiness, jealousy, or revenge.

Here are some you might like to try:

I am kind.
I am intelligent.
I am loving.
I am inspiring.

So much of our day is consumed with obsessing over details, which then leads to stress, but if you remind yourself of the greater and more important affirmations, then everything else will take care of itself. There's no way we can predict all the things that we might be faced with throughout the day, but we can remind ourselves to be loving, kind, strong, and great. It will put you in a far more powerful place to deal with whatever comes your way each day. Be the manifestation of those things. That is very powerful.

Is meditation important?

There is so much in this world that we don't know or understand. Our awareness allows us to see only so much, and we can see only what we can comprehend. If all we are doing is focusing on our job, our appearance, our income, and our relationships, then we are asleep to our own deeper dimensions. Meditation and sleep are like brain retreats, allowing us to achieve a stillness that is available to all of us if we choose to reach for it. Meditation nourishes and unwinds the mind and body, which is beneficial not only for us individually but also for those around us. For me, meditation is like having a massage for the soul. A 2009 Stanford study showed that a six-week meditation course helped people who had trouble sleeping to fall asleep twice as quickly. The science proves it: meditation helps us sleep, and together the two can totally transform our overall wellbeing.

The Roman emperor Marcus Aurelius wrote in his book *Meditations*, "People look for retreats for themselves, in the country, by the coast, or in the hills when it's possible to retreat into yourself any time you want. There is nowhere that a person can find a more peaceful or trouble-free retreat than in his own mind." Meditation doesn't mean you have to become a monk on top of a mountain; it's just about dedicating time to yourself when you can focus on your breath and let your thoughts float in and out. There is no one way to meditate, and these days there are endless apps, books, and courses to help you find what's right for you.

Can I afford not to meditate?

I had a conversation about this with a great friend whom I deeply admire; he has meditated for many years and found great positives from it. Over time, he's learned to take that feeling he got from practicing meditation and fuse it into his daily life. So, rather than experiencing "Stress-stress-stress. Pause for meditation. Stress-stress-stress," he has found a way to feel genuinely happy and peaceful all day long and integrate the benefits of meditation into every minute of every day. I try to do that in my life, too. Meditation is amazing, but rather than relying on it for downtime, inject that ease you get from meditation into your everyday life, into every minute of every day, until it becomes part of who you actually are.

Eventually, your whole life should be a meditation on happiness, joy, courage, kindness and all of the things that are important to you.

How can I relax to recharge?

Being relaxed doesn't have to mean that you're sleepy or lazy or not getting things done. For instance, in a tennis match, the player who wins the tournament is the one who stays calm and focused. It's the same with fighting (one of the most stressful situations you could put yourself in, with not one moment when you can afford to be lazy—otherwise, you lose): the fighter who can relax through it, remaining calm and serene, is usually the winner. That's what I've learned from jiu-jitsu. It's like quicksand—the more you struggle and stress, the more difficult the situation becomes, while having a sense of ease and learning to relax is the way to win. It's like being in *The Matrix*! When I fight against someone who isn't as relaxed as I am, that's when I win. I'm not naturally talented or a phenomenal athlete, but I win competitions because I can stay calm. It's the same in your everyday life. Some people don't feel they are working hard unless they are stressed, and they fear people won't respect what they say unless they deliver it in a shouty, stressed-out, urgent way—but it's just not true. People respond best to calmness, and it shines through. Finding peace in the chaos is true mastery and yet so achievable.

Remember the words of one of my favorite poems: *If* by Rudyard Kipling.

If you can keep your head when all about you
Are losing theirs and blaming it on you,
If you can trust yourself when all men doubt you,
But make allowance for their doubting too;
If you can wait and not be tired by waiting,
[...]
Yours is the Earth and everything that's in it,
And—which is more—you'll be a Man, my son!

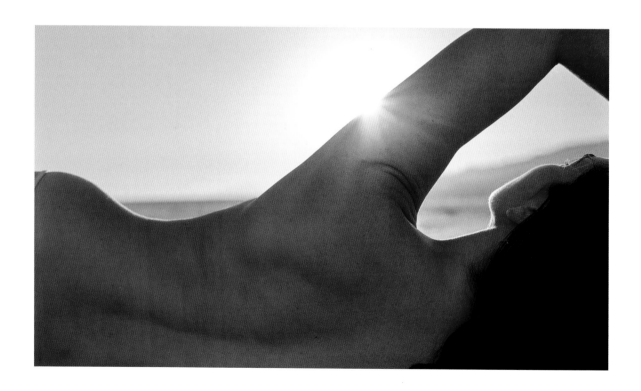

Bodyism Meditations

Here are some meditations for you to add to your morning, day, or winding-down routine:

On-the-Go Meditation

This is one to practice when you are out and about. Sometimes we just need a few minutes to reset and this meditation will do exactly that.

Focus on all your senses, with no judgment.

Be completely present to where you are. Notice the color of the trees, the wind in your face, the smells surrounding you, and the feeling of your feet in your shoes. Rather than judge, notice the sensations and be present in the moment. Any thoughts that drop in, accept them and let them pass.

Be in the present moment, right here, right now.

Power of the Breath Meditation

Always come back to the power of your breath; it can totally transform your mental and physical wellbeing. Full, deep breathing can lower tension and stress and will help you totally relax.

The object of this meditation is to learn how to get in touch with the rhythm of your breathing and learn to breathe in a relaxed, unstressed way. It can be practiced in any position, but it's best to start off by lying on your back, with your knees bent.

This meditation can be practiced daily, either first thing or as part of your winding-down routine. You can do it almost anywhere; it's a relaxation tool that you can use any time you need it.

Caution: Some people get dizzy the first few times they practice this, but it's just your body adjusting.

Place one hand on your stomach and your other hand on your chest. Notice how your hands move as you breathe in and out.

Practice breathing so that the hand on your tummy rises when you inhale and the hand on your chest stays still. Inhale for five seconds through your nose, pause for three seconds, and exhale for five seconds through your mouth. Keep your shoulders relaxed throughout.

When you have noticed your stomach rising and falling a few times, add the second step to your breathing: inhale first into your stomach, and then continue inhaling into your chest. You should feel the hand on your chest rising, too.

As you exhale, feel the tension leaving your body as you become more and more relaxed.

Practice this for five minutes. Notice the constant movement of your breathing, like waves coming in and out.

Recharge Meditation

This is a great meditation to do first thing. It always energizes me for the day ahead; make it a habit.

Begin in a comfortable seated position, with your spine supported and your palms resting, either face-up or down, on your knees. If you can't sit on the floor, a chair is fine, or even lying down is okay—as long as the spine is straight.

Turn your attention to your breath. Notice your inhalation and exhalation.

What is the rhythm of your breathing? A stressed state will often cause a faster inhalation and an unfulfilled exhalation. A slow and calm exhalation stimulates the parasympathetic nervous system, increasing your ability to digest and detoxify. It is also on the exhalation that we release toxins in the form of carbon dioxide.

Every breath you take is recharging you. Start to count with each breath.

Inhale for three seconds. Hold it for three seconds. Exhale for six seconds.

Repeat for eight rounds and count the rounds on your hand by touching your thumb to each finger as you move to the next one.

At the top of each inhalation, in your head repeat the mantra, "I am recharged," and, on each exhalation, visualize all the toxins and tensions leaving your body.

Notice how you feel after these lengthened breaths.

Slowly open your eyes.

Relaxed Meditation

We do not become stronger, fitter, or leaner when we train; instead, the transformation actually happens when we relax. If we can't relax, our training and nutritious diet will not be supported by the body. This meditation is about relaxation.

Begin in a comfortable seated position, with your spine supported and palms resting, either face-up or down, on your knees. If you can't sit on the floor, a chair or lying down is fine too—as long as the spine is straight.

Turn your attention to your breath. Notice your inhalation and exhalation. What is the rhythm of your breathing? Relax your body by lengthening the breath.

Every breath you take is relaxing you. Start to count with each breath.

Inhale for three seconds. Hold it for three seconds. Exhale for six seconds.

Repeat for eight rounds, counting the rounds on your hand by touching your thumb to each finger as you go.

Once you have relaxed the body, repeat this mantra in synchronization with your breath:

Inhale: "I am . . ."

Exhale: "relaxed."

Repeat three times.

Open your eyes slowly. Take a moment to notice the connection between your body and mind.

Your Unique Meditation

This time, you have the opportunity to choose your own mantra. Choose a mantra that suits your current life situation. Think of what your body, mind, and spirit need most and affirm it with your mantra and breath. Add this into your day whenever you need to refocus, or when you just need some extra support.

Begin in a comfortable seated position, with your spine supported and palms resting, either face-up or down, on your knees. Again, if you can't sit on the floor, a chair or even lying down is fine—as long as the spine is straight.

Turn your attention to your breath. Notice your inhalation and exhalation. What is the rhythm of your breathing?

Every breath you take is cleansing you. Count with each breath.

Inhale for three seconds. Hold it for three seconds. Exhale for six seconds.

Repeat for three rounds—counting the rounds, as before, by touching your thumb to each finger as you move to the next one. Once you have relaxed your body, repeat the mantra of your choice in synchronization with your breath:

Inhale: "I am . . . "

Exhale: ". . . happy" / "calm" / "free" / "open" / "organized" / "capable" / "beautiful" / "energized." The choice is yours.

Connect to the feeling of that particular affirmation and let it fill you with eagerness for your life.

Repeat eight times.

Open your eyes slowly. Take a moment to notice the connection to your body and mind.

Did You Know? An entire industry has been created to fuel a population living with continuous exhaustion. In the US, more than 55 million prescriptions for sleeping pills were written in 2014 alone, with sales exceeding $1 billion. Jerome Siegel, director of UCLA's Center for Sleep Research, explained that, in the near future, "people will look back on the sleeping-pill era as we now look back on the acceptance of cigarette smoking." The chronic use of sleeping pills is a total disaster. The amount of money, time, and brainpower that goes into them is not solving any problems. These pills do not offer a magic solution to giving us a good night's sleep; they just distract us from the benefits of real, restorative sleep.

Here are just some of the side effects of the sleeping pills: anxiety; bladder pain; bloody or cloudy urine; change in walking and balance; chills; cold sweats; cough; crying; decreased awareness or responsiveness; delusions; dementia; depersonalization; dizziness; dry mouth; dysphoria; euphoria; fainting; frequent urge to urinate; hyperventilation; irregular heartbeats; irritability; light-headedness when getting up from a lying or sitting position; lower back or side pain; painful urination (burning, itching, numbness, prickling); paranoia, "pins and needles"; rapidly changing moods; severe sleepiness; shakiness in the legs, arms, hands, or feet; shortness of breath; violent behaviors.

A study from the Scripps Research Institute, led by Dr. Daniel Kripke, found that those who had taken 18 sleeping tablets in a year had a risk of death three times higher during the two-and-half-year study than those who had not taken any pills. I could write an endless list of the links between disease and sleeping pills. They're linked to cancer, infertility, dementia, the list goes on. Reaching for a sleeping pill is the opposite of being kind to yourself.

BODYISM TWO-WEEK BLUEPRINT

This is your opportunity to elevate your health and create a beautiful, vibrant, and energized body. When you embrace this plan, you will begin to learn the many different ways in which your body is speaking to you. You can let go of old, unhealthy, and unhelpful habits. Once you have mastered the art of listening to your body, you will never need another diet book, exercise plan, app, or any other "guide" again because the answers will come from the only expert you will ever need—you. This is the first step you can make to be kind to yourself.

WEEK ONE

Monday

Mindset: Say your affirmations and choose one meditation to fit into your day.

Movement: Prehab Circuit, 2x Perfect Posture Circuit, Quick Cardio Burst, 2x Perky Butt Circuit, Quick Cardio Burst, Regenerate Circuit

Action: Drink 8 cups of water/herbal tea throughout your day.

Nutrition: Breakfast—The Protein Wrap (page 108)
Lunch—Bowl of your choice (pages 102–129)
Shake—Body Brilliance Shake (page 218)
Dinner—Zucchini Lasagna (page 142)

Sleep: Think/write/speak aloud your gratitude journal (page 82). Wind down by 10 p.m.

Tuesday

Mindset: Say your affirmations and choose one meditation to fit into your day.

Movement: Prehab Circuit, 2x Long Lean Legs, Quick Cardio Burst, 2x Flat-tummy Circuit, Quick Cardio Burst, Regenerate Circuit

Action: Remember to chew your food.

Nutrition: Breakfast—Simply Granola, with nut milk and a sprinkling of berries (page 102)
Lunch—Alkalizing Supergreen Soup (page 137) with a side of your choice
Shake—Beauty Food Shake (page 216)
Dinner—Turmeric Dal (page 147) with some greens

Sleep: Think/write/speak aloud your gratitude journal (page 82). Wind down by 10 p.m.

Wednesday

Mindset: Say your affirmations and choose one meditation to fit into your day.

Movement: 30-minute walk/yoga class/try a new class with a friend.

Action: Add a portion of greens to one of your meals today.

Nutrition: Breakfast—The Egg Bowl. (page 110)
Lunch—Bowl of your choice (pages 120–129)
Shake—Berry Burn Shake (page 219)
Dinner—Poached Coconut Chicken and Cauli-rice (page 160) with greens. Note: make extra chicken for tomorrow.

Sleep: Think/write/speak aloud your gratitude journal (page 82). Wind down by 10 p.m.

Thursday

Mindset: Say your affirmations and choose one meditation to fit into your day.

Movement: Prehab Circuit, 2x Perky Butt Circuit, Quick Cardio Burst, 2x Long Lean Legs, Quick Cardio Burst, Regenerate Circuit

Action: Do a random act of kindness today; it's the best way to create power in your own life.

Nutrition: Breakfast—The Protein Wrap (page 108)
Lunch—Leftover Coconut Chicken (page 160) with Kabbouleh (page 134)
Shake—Ultimate Clean Shake (page 216)
Dinner—Ultimate Fish Pie (page 143) with greens

Sleep: Think/write/speak aloud your gratitude journal (page 82). Wind down by 10 p.m.

Friday

Mindset: Say your affirmations and choose one meditation to fit into your day.

Movement: Prehab Circuit, 2x Perfect Posture Circuit, Quick Cardio Burst, 2x Flat-tummy Circuit, Quick Cardio Burst, Regenerate Circuit

Action: Commit to switching your phone off at 9 p.m. tonight.

Nutrition: Breakfast—Bircher Muesli (page 101)
Lunch—Bowl of your choice (pages 120–129)
Shake—Chai Cashew Mylk (page 220)
Dinner—Keralan Fish Curry (page 161) with veggies of your choice

Sleep: Think/write/speak aloud your gratitude journal (page 82). Wind down by 10 p.m.

Saturday

Mindset: Say your affirmations and choose one meditation to fit into your day.

Movement: Prehab Circuit, 2x Perky Butt Circuit, Quick Cardio Burst, 2x Flat-tummy Circuit, Quick Cardio Burst, Regenerate Circuit

Action: Tell someone you love them today. This may sound corny, but it's one of the most powerful things you can do.

Nutrition: Breakfast—Brunchy Baked Eggs (page 114)
Lunch—Chickpea Dosa Wrap (page 133)
Shake—Body Brilliance Shake (page 96)
Dinner—Perfect Roast Chicken (page 162) with a side of your choice and some greens

Sleep: Think/write/speak aloud your gratitude journal (page 82). Wind down by 10 p.m.

Sunday

Mindset: Say your affirmations and choose one meditation to fit into your day.

Movement: Rest and try to get a massage.

Action: Remember to chill today.

Nutrition: Breakfast—Buckwheat, Egg, Carrot, and Mushroom Crêpes (page 117)
Lunch—Turmeric, Sweet Potato, Ginger, and Coconut Soup (page 138) with buckwheat and radish salad
Snack—Bodyism Cookie (page 176) Remember portion control, here—you can always have cookies again.
Dinner—Bodyism Frittata (page 136) Note: make enough for breakfast tomorrow.

Sleep: Think/write/speak aloud your gratitude journal (page 82). Wind down by 10 p.m.

WEEK TWO

Monday

Mindset: Say your affirmations and choose one meditation to fit into your day.

Movement: Prehab Circuit, 2x Perfect Posture Circuit, Quick Cardio Burst, 2x Long Lean Legs, Quick Cardio Burst, Regenerate Circuit

Action: Spend five minutes focusing on your breath.

Nutrition: Breakfast—Leftover Bodyism Frittata (page 136)
Lunch—Bowl of your choice (pages 120–129)
Shake—Body Brilliance Shake (page 218)
Dinner—Perfect Roast Chicken, with a side of your choice (page 162) Note: make sure you cook enough chicken so you'll have leftovers.

Sleep: Think/write/speak aloud your gratitude journal (page 82). Wind down by 10 p.m.

Tuesday

Mindset: Say your affirmations and choose one meditation to fit into your day.

Movement: Prehab Circuit, 2x Perfect Posture Circuit, Quick Cardio Burst, 2x Perky Butt Circuit, Quick Cardio Burst, Regenerate Circuit

Action: Say thank you ... It's the fastest way to get yourself into a state of gratitude, which is one of the happiest, most wonderful states of being.

Nutrition: Breakfast—Three-Grain Oatmeal (page 100)
Lunch—Chicken Pho (page 167)
Shake—Ultimate Clean Shake (page 216)
Dinner—Tuna Poké Bowl (page 154)

Sleep: Think/write/speak aloud your gratitude journal (page 82). Wind down by 10 p.m.

Wednesday

Mindset: Say your affirmations and choose one meditation to fit into your day.

Movement: 30-minute walk/a dance class/a boxing class—try something new!

Action: Drink 8 cups of water/herbal tea throughout your day.

Nutrition: Breakfast—Açai Bowl (page 96)
Lunch—Bowl of your choice (pages 120–129)
Shake—Beauty Food Shake (page 216)
Dinner—Turmeric Dal (page 147) Note: make enough for tomorrow.

Sleep: Think/write/speak aloud your gratitude journal (page 82). Wind down by 10 p.m.

Thursday

Mindset: Say your affirmations and choose one meditation to fit into your day.

Movement: Prehab Circuit, 2x Flat-tummy Circuit, Quick Cardio Burst, 2x Long Lean Legs, Quick Cardio Burst, Regenerate Circuit

Action: Choose to be more powerful than all of your excuses.

Nutrition: Breakfast—Leftover Turmeric Dal (page 147) with a fried egg on top!
Lunch—Alkalizing Supergreen Soup (page 137)
Shake—Berry Burn Shake (page 219)
Dinner—Sexy Stir-Fry (page 157) with a protein of your choice (chicken, lamb, fish)

Sleep: Think/write/speak aloud your gratitude journal (page 82). Wind down by 10 p.m.

Friday

Mindset: Say your affirmations and choose one meditation to fit into your day.

Movement: Prehab Circuit, 2x Perfect Posture Circuit, Quick Cardio Burst, 2x Flat-tummy Circuit, Quick Cardio Burst, Regenerate Circuit

Action: Remind yourself of your "why," if you are tempted to fall back into old habits.

Nutrition: Breakfast—Bircher Muesli (page 101)
Lunch—Bowl of your choice (pages 120–129)
Shake—Body Brilliance Shake (page 218)
Dinner—Moroccan Tagine (page 152) Note: make enough for tomorrow.

Sleep: Think/write/speak aloud your gratitude journal (page 82). Wind down by 10 p.m.

Saturday

Mindset: Say your affirmations and choose one meditation to fit into your day.

Movement: Prehab Circuit, 2x Perky Butt Circuit, Quick Cardio Burst, 2x Flat-tummy Circuit, Quick Cardio Burst, Regenerate Circuit

Action: Practice being present; have a conversation with someone, don't have your phone anywhere near, and listen genuinely to him or her.

Nutrition: Breakfast—Indian Spiced Eggs (page 107)
Lunch—Turmeric, Sweet Potato, Ginger, and Coconut Soup (page 138) with buckwheat and radish salad
Shake—Beauty Food Shake (page 216)
Dinner—Leftover Moroccan Tagine (page 152)

Sleep: Think/write/speak aloud your gratitude journal (page 82). Wind down by 10 p.m.

Sunday

Mindset: Say your affirmations and choose one meditation to fit into your day.

Movement: Rest and try to get a massage.

Action: Be proud of yourself, enjoy the moment, take on the lessons from your body and your experience from the past two weeks, and allow them to strengthen you for the future.

Nutrition: Breakfast—Chocolate Soup (page 99) because it's Sunday!
Lunch—Miso Shrimp and Eggplant Salad (page 132) and a slice of Honey Cake (page 202)
Shake—Chai Cashew Mylk (page 220)
Dinner—The Perfect Burger (page 164) and Sweet Potato Wedges (page 191)

Sleep: Think/write/speak aloud your gratitude journal (see page 82). Wind down by 10 p.m.

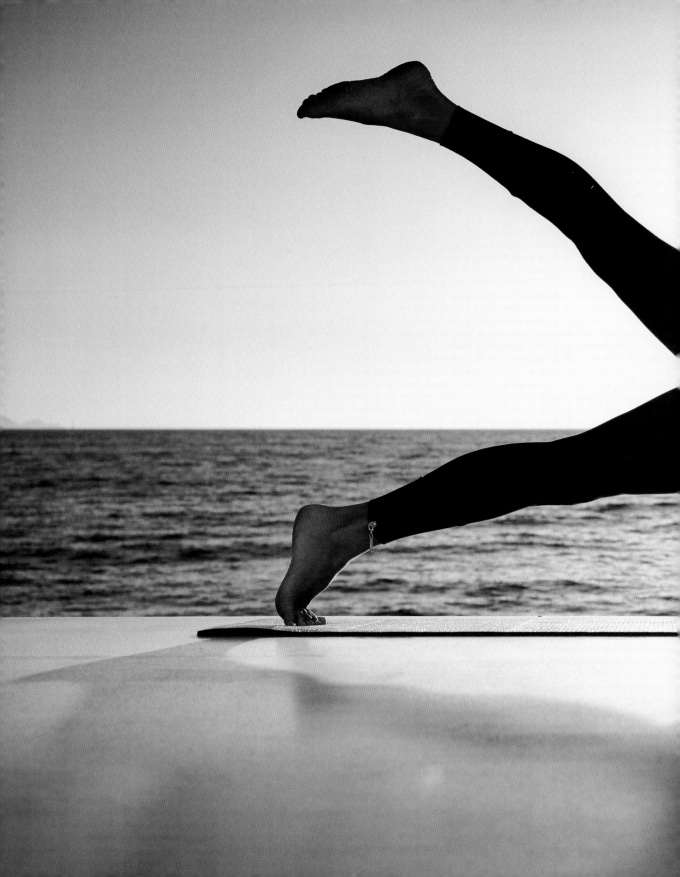

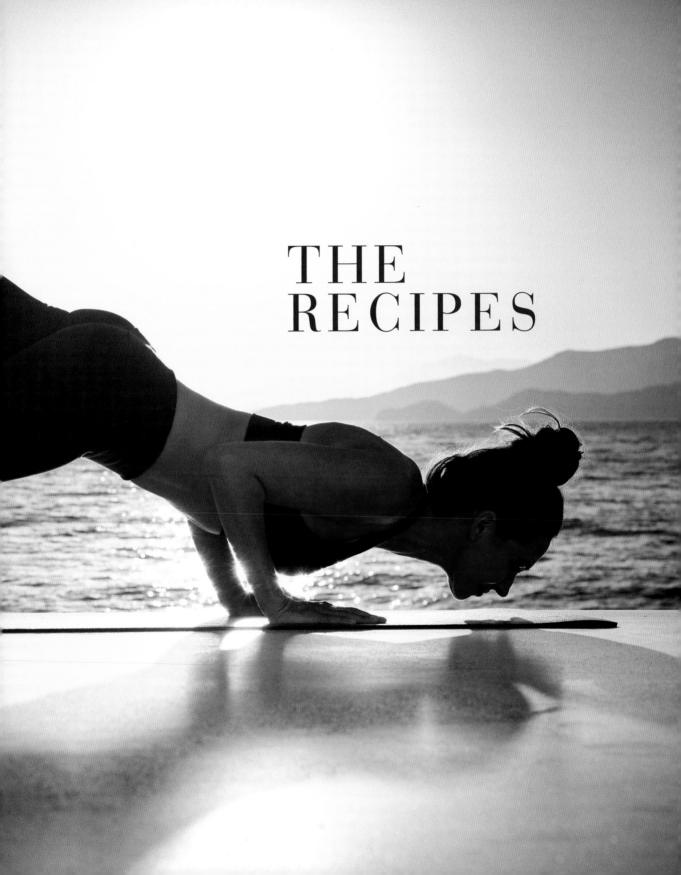

THE
RECIPES

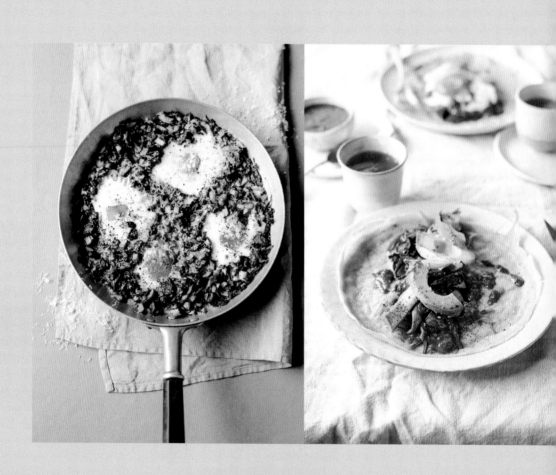

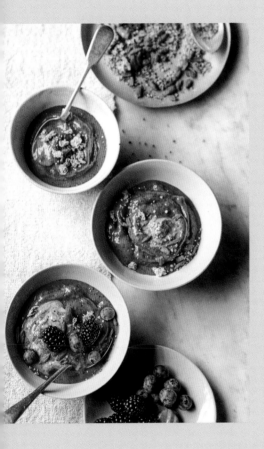

BREAKFAST

Açai Bowl

Chocolate Soup

Three-Grain Oatmeal

Bircher Muesli

Simply Granola

Protein Pancakes

Chai Carrot Chew-Chew

Almond and Coconut Pancakes with Roasted Spiced Peaches

Indian Spiced Eggs

The Protein Wrap

The Egg Bowl

Avocado, Tomato, and Chile Salsa with Quinoa Bread

Healthy Breakfast Hash

Brunchy Baked Eggs

Buckwheat, Egg, Carrot, and Mushroom Crêpes

AÇAI BOWL

Açai is one of the most nutritious fruits in the world. We blend ours with one of the Bodyism supplements to increase the protein content in each bowl and to make it even more delicious.

Our açai supplier, Rayder, is an activist for preventing deforestation in the Amazon, and açai is one of the only no-timber products to come from the rainforest. So, make sure you choose high-quality frozen açai (you can find it in health stores or online) and feel proud that you are helping to save the planet and looking after your body, too. If you don't have the Bodyism supplements, substitute them for a tablespoon of hemp seeds.

serves 2
3½ oz frozen açai pulp
half a frozen banana
1 scoop Bodyism Body Brilliance or Bodyism
    Protein Excellence
¼ cup almond milk
½ cup frozen mixed berries

for the toppings
2 tbsp almond butter
2 tbsp Simply Granola (see page 102)
2 tbsp fresh berries
any other superfood you'd like: goji berries,
    hemp seeds, bee pollen, coconut flakes,
    or chia seeds

1. Put the açai, banana, Bodyism supplement, and almond milk into a blender. Blend it up until all the açai is mixed (if there are any unblended pieces left, then add more almond milk).

2. Spoon into bowls. Add the toppings equally into each bowl. Start with the almond butter, then granola and finally sprinkle with berries and any other superfood you want!

Top Tip Texture is everything. Aim for an ice-cream consistency, not a smoothie —it is an art!

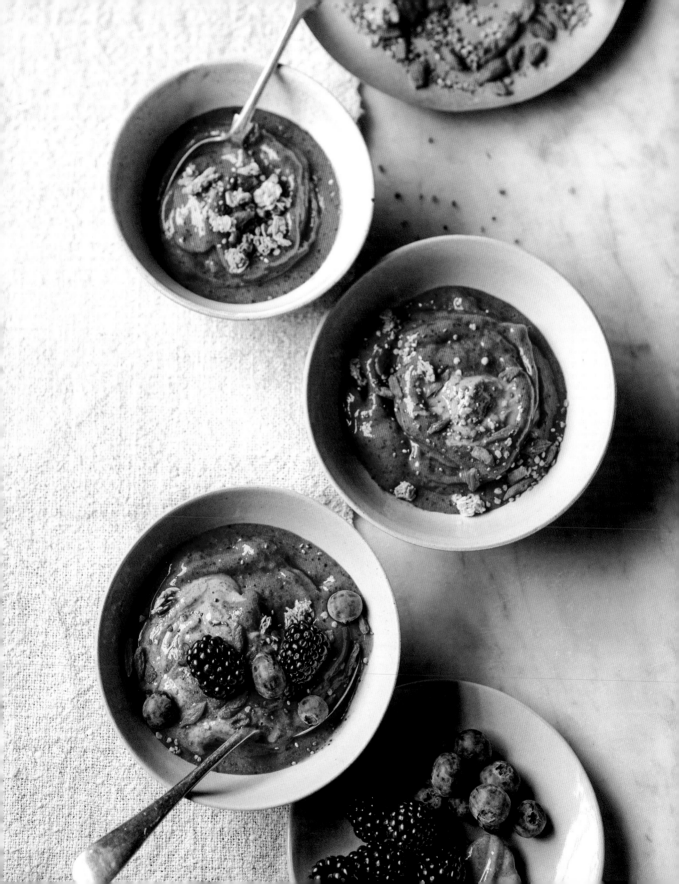

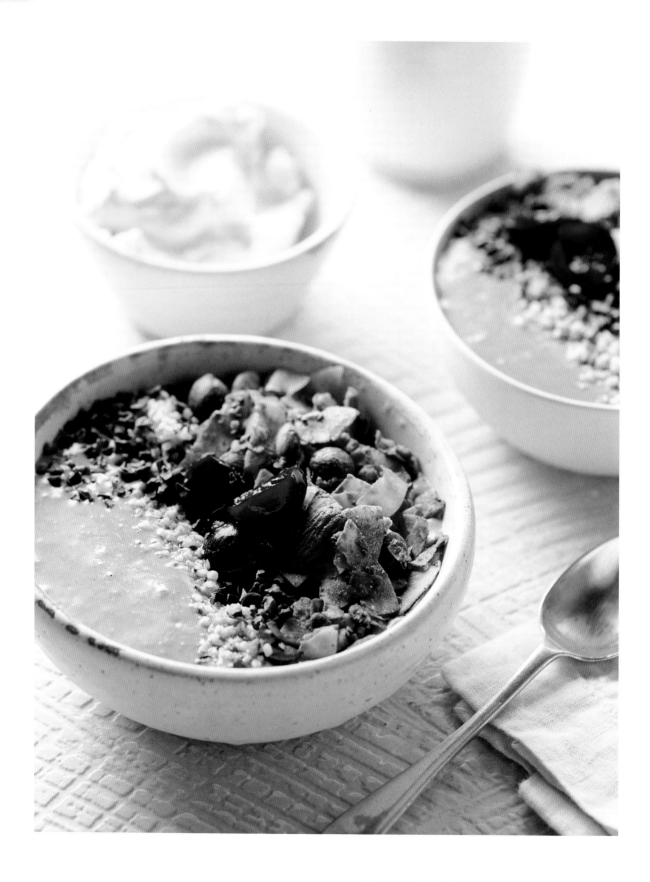

CHOCOLATE SOUP

Otherwise known as "Soup of Eternal Blissful Love." I fell in love with Chrissy while eating a chocolate soup, so now I've come up with a healthy version that nourishes your body, helps you burn fat, and guarantees that you will fall in love with the first person you see after eating it ... It's a delicious nutrient boost for both your body and your taste buds.

   If you don't have the Bodyism supplements, get them! Or, if not, then add a tablespoon of hemp seeds to get an extra boost of protein.

serves 2

2 cups unsweetened almond milk
½ cup coconut yogurt
½ tsp vanilla extract
2 bananas, frozen
3 tbsp cacao powder
3 tbsp hazelnut butter (or another nut butter
   of your choice)
handful of frozen spinach
1 scoop Bodyism Protein Excellence
   (optional)
1 scoop Bodyism Body Brilliance (optional)

1. Put all the ingredients into a blender and blend
   until smooth.

2. Add any topping you like!

for the toppings (per serving)

1 tbsp cacao nibs
1 tbsp Simply Granola (page 102)
1 tsp hazelnut butter
1 tbsp hemp seeds
6 frozen cherries
1 tbsp coconut milk (drizzled on the top)

Top Tip This also tastes delicious frozen — it is the Bodyism version of chocolate ice cream!

THREE-GRAIN OATMEAL

If you can, try to soak the grains for this recipe overnight. Soaking them makes them easier to digest and quicker to cook in the morning.

serves 2

¼ cup rolled gluten-free oats
½ oz buckwheat flakes
⅓ oz buckwheat groats
1 cup water
½ cup almond milk
1 tbsp chia seeds
generous pinch of salt
1 tsp ground cinnamon
1 scoop Bodyism Protein Excellence

for the toppings

2 tbsp coconut yogurt
3½ oz sugar-free strawberry jam
2 tbsp almond flakes, toasted
2 tbsp blueberries

1. Soak the oats, buckwheat flakes, and groats in water overnight. Use just enough water to cover the grains.

2. Put the soaked grains, water, and almond milk in a saucepan. Add the chia seeds and stir. Bring slowly to a boil. Turn down the heat and add the salt, cinnamon, and Protein Excellence. Stir well until you achieve the consistency you want.

3. Divide between two bowls, add a spoon of coconut yogurt and strawberry jam to each, then sprinkle with almond flakes and blueberries and enjoy!

Top Tip My little boy, Leo, loves a chocolate version. Add in a scoop of Body Brilliance, one teaspoon of almond butter and one teaspoon of cacao.

BIRCHER MUESLI

This is such a wholesome breakfast and is always one of my go-to recipes in the winter months when I'm craving something that is going to keep me feeling full up till lunch. I love to mix the Bodyism Protein Excellence supplement into this recipe and eat it straight after a morning workout. Feel free to experiment with the flavor—try adding cacao or ginger or swap the fruit for whatever is in season.

serves 2
½ cup rolled oats
½ cup cooked quinoa
1 tbsp chia seeds
1 tbsp sunflower seeds
2 tbsp shredded coconut
1 tbsp goji berries
½ tsp ground cinnamon
½ tsp ground ginger
1 tsp vanilla extract
½ cup blueberries
½ cup coconut water
¼ cup coconut milk
½ cup coconut yogurt
1 scoop Bodyism Protein Excellence
   (optional)

for the topping
½ cup coconut yogurt
handful of blueberries or stewed apple
handful of toasted coconut flakes
handful of toasted pistachios, shelled
drizzle of maple syrup (optional)

1. In a bowl, mix the oats, cooked quinoa, chia seeds, sunflower seeds, shredded coconut, goji berries, cinnamon, ginger, and vanilla extract.

2. In a small bowl, mash the blueberries slightly so they release their delicious juice and then stir them into the muesli.

3. Add the coconut water, milk, and yogurt and stir well. If you are adding the supplement, stir it in here too. Stir to combine well, cover, and leave in the fridge overnight.

4. In the morning, divide the mixture into two bowls. Top with a spoon of coconut yogurt, berries or stewed apple, some coconut flakes, pistachios, and, if you'd like, a small drizzle of maple syrup.

Top Tip Double the recipe and keep the mixture in a jar so that you have a delicious quick breakfast for the week.

SIMPLY GRANOLA

Granola is often the "Mean Girls" of breakfast. It's basically pretending to be your friend, but actually it's making you fat. Store-bought granola is so often full of sugar in all its different forms—whether it's dates or brown-rice syrup—whatever it is, it will be hidden in there. This granola is genuinely healthy and can be eaten regularly with love and joy.

serves 6

3 cups rolled oats
2 cups buckwheat flakes
⅓ cup buckwheat groats
¼ cup pecans, chopped
¼ cup cashews (or a nut of your choice), chopped
¼ cup pumpkin seeds
⅛ cup sunflower seeds
2 tbsp flaxseeds
½ cup coconut flakes
4 tbsp coconut oil
2 tbsp ground cinnamon
3 tsp vanilla powder
1 tsp Himalayan pink salt

1. Preheat the oven to 375°F and line 2 baking sheets with parchment paper.

2. Put the oats, buckwheat flakes and groats, nuts, seeds, and coconut into a big mixing bowl. Mix well.

3. In a saucepan, melt the coconut oil. Take the oil off the heat and add the cinnamon, vanilla, and salt. Mix well.

4. Pour the oil mixture into the mixing bowl and stir well.

5. Spread the mixture evenly on the baking sheets. Using a spatula, push the mixture firmly onto the sheet. Bake for 20 minutes in the preheated oven, using the spatula to turn the granola mixture over halfway through baking.

6. Leave to cool in the baking sheets. Once at room temperature, pour the granola into an airtight container. Enjoy this with rice milk or coconut yogurt for breakfast, or sprinkle over Chocolate Soup (page 99) or Açai Bowl (page 96).

Top Tip Remember the granola will continue to cook once it's out of the oven so don't let it burn!

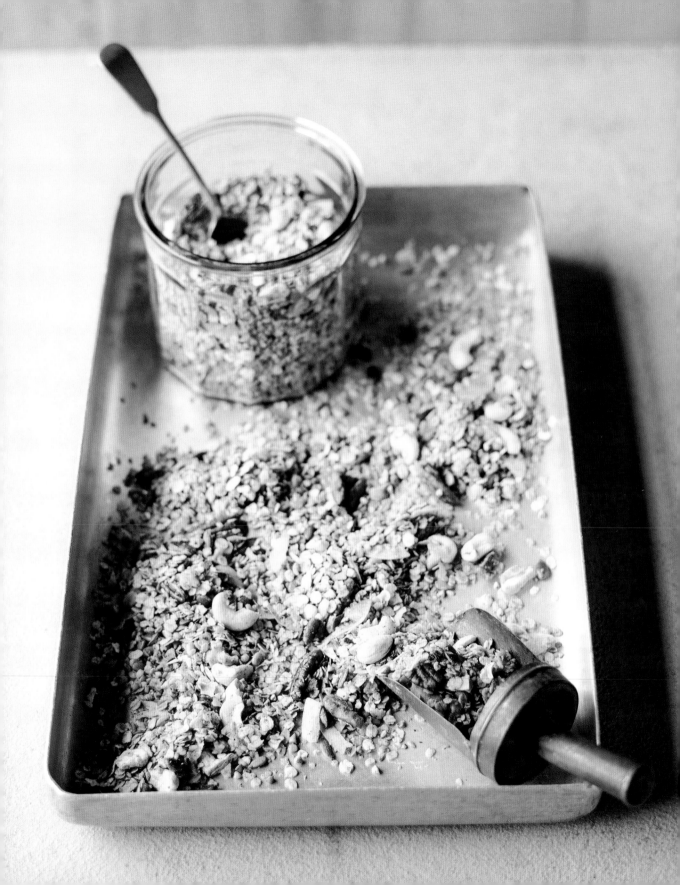

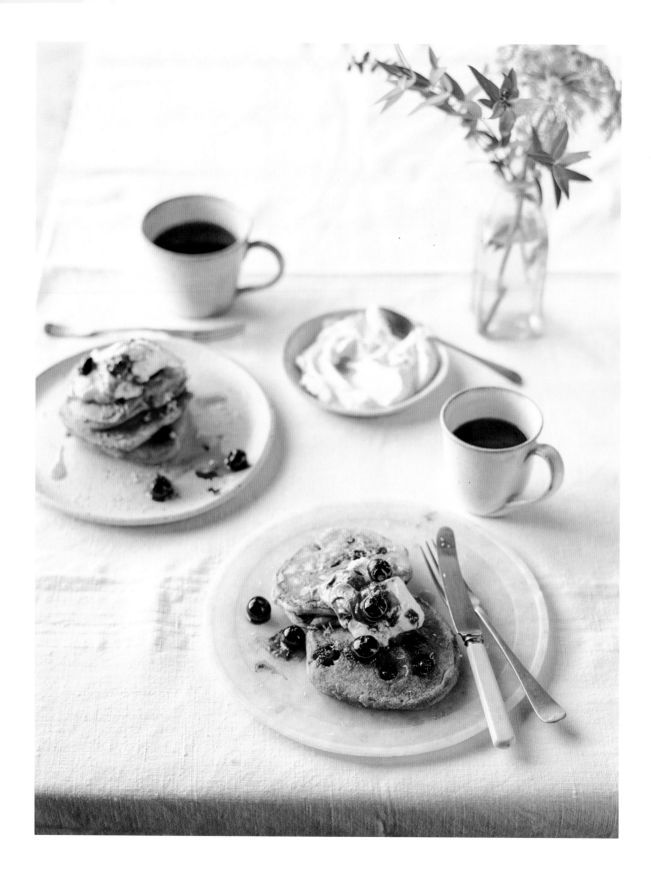

PROTEIN PANCAKES

This pancake is too legit to quit. It's an OG (original gangsta) of the Bodyism world. Delicious and loved by everyone—children, grumpy husbands—and, if you don't tell anyone it's healthy, they'll just keep asking for more..

serves 2 (makes a stack of 6)
1 banana, sliced
2 organic, free-range eggs
1¾ scoops Bodyism Protein Excellence
pinch of ground cinnamon
¼ tsp baking soda
zest of 1 lemon
2 tbsp almond milk
1 tsp coconut oil
handful of blueberries (optional)

for the toppings
4 tbsp coconut yogurt
1 tsp almond butter
2 tbsp fresh berries

1. Put the banana, eggs, Protein Excellence, cinnamon, baking soda, lemon zest, and almond milk into a blender. Blend it up until it is well mixed.

2. Add the oil to a skillet and place over medium heat, spreading the oil around the pan.

3. Add 2 tablespoons of pancake batter into the pan. Sprinkle with blueberries if you like. Leave to cook for 1–2 minutes before flipping and then cook for another 1–2 minutes on the other side. Do this until all the mixture is used up.

4. Stack the pancakes and top with coconut yogurt, almond butter, and fresh berries.

CHAI CARROT CHEW-CHEW

This is traditionally an Indian dessert; however, I think it makes an impressive grain-free breakfast. You'll notice ghee enhances the sweetness of the carrots.

serves 2
2 large carrots
2 tsp coconut oil or ghee
1 cup coconut milk
1 tbsp golden raisins
1 tsp ground cardamom
1 tsp ground cinnamon
handful of pistachios, roughly chopped
1 tbsp chia seeds

1. Start by washing and coarsely grating the carrots, then set aside.

2. Heat the oil or ghee in a small saucepan over low heat and add the grated carrots. Cook for 5 minutes, until the carrots smell fragrant.

3. Add the milk, golden raisins, cardamom, and cinnamon and stir over low heat for 10 minutes, or until the liquid is absorbed. Serve with the chopped pistachios and chia seeds.

ALMOND AND COCONUT PANCAKES WITH ROASTED, SPICED PEACHES

This is mouth-wateringly good—and, what's more, it's not rammed with refined sugar, chemicals, salt, or any of the other junk that makes you feel less than what you deserve. There is honey in it, so don't have it every day, but when you do, enjoy it.

serves 4

for the peaches

12 peaches

1 tsp pumpkin pie spice

1 tsp ground ginger

1 tbsp organic honey (optional)

1 tsp grated orange zest

2 tbsp orange juice

for the pancakes

¼ cup coconut flour

1 cup ground almonds

1 scoop Bodyism Protein Excellence (optional)

1 tsp ground ginger

1 tsp ground cinnamon

1½ tsp baking powder

4 organic, free-range eggs

1 cup coconut milk

1 tsp vanilla extract

1 tbsp maple syrup (optional)

2 tbsp coconut oil

1. Preheat the oven to 350°F and line a baking sheet with parchment paper.

2. Cut the peaches into quarters, discarding the pits.

3. Mix together the spice, ginger, honey, orange zest, and juice. Place two thirds of the peach quarters on the baking sheet and drizzle the liquid over them.

4. Roast for 15 minutes in the preheated oven and then leave to cool. Place the cooked peaches in a bowl, reserving the juice in a separate bowl.

5. Place the remaining uncooked peaches and the juice from the cooked peaches in a food processor and blend. Pour into a small bowl and set aside.

6. To make the pancakes, mix the flour, ground almonds, Protein Excellence, ground ginger, cinnamon, and baking powder in a large bowl. In a separate bowl, mix the eggs, coconut milk, vanilla extract, and maple syrup (if using) together. Slowly beat this into the dry mixture to make a batter.

7. Set a small nonstick skillet over medium heat. Add the oil and, once melted, drop a large spoonful of pancake batter into the hot pan, spreading it around the base. Cook for 1 minute, then flip and cook until golden brown. Using a spatula, lift out of the pan and set aside until all 4 pancakes are cooked.

8. Reheat the peaches and serve on top of the pancakes with a drizzle of the sauce.

INDIAN SPICED EGGS

If you're feeling adventurous and want to spice up your scrambled eggs, this is the recipe for you. Turmeric is an incredible anti-inflammatory, so not only is this delicious, but it's really good for your health, too.

serves 4

1 tbsp coconut oil
1 small red onion, finely chopped
2 garlic cloves, crushed
1 green chile, seeded and finely chopped
¼ tsp ground cumin
¼ tsp garam masala
¼ tsp ground turmeric
4 large tomatoes, seeded and finely chopped
8 organic, free-range eggs, beaten
good pinch of salt and pepper
1 tbsp cilantro, finely chopped (plus extra for serving)

1. Heat a large skillet over low to medium heat and add the oil. Fry the onion, garlic, and chile until the onion is soft (approximately 5 minutes). Add the spices and stir for another 1–2 minutes.

2. Add the tomatoes to the pan and stir. Leave to sauté for 30 seconds.

3. Pour in the eggs and lower the heat. Season with salt and pepper. Stir slowly to scramble the eggs as they cook. Remove from the heat when they are still a little runny and then stir in the cilantro. Continue to stir for another minute.

4. Serve with a Chickpea Dosa Wrap (page 133) or a slice of sourdough toast. Garnish with a sprig of cilantro before serving.

Did You Know? Turmeric becomes a superhero antioxidant only when it is activated with pepper.

THE PROTEIN WRAP

This wrap is so versatile. We always blend leftover vegetables in the blender before adding them into the egg mix. They look so bright and delicious with beets! Charlotte loves that she can have a pink breakfast. (We always make this when she has friends over.)

Also, we make up a big batch of them at the start of the week and then just heat them up in a skillet over the next few days.

serves 1
1 organic, free-range egg
1 tsp dried mixed herbs
1 small pre-cooked beet
pinch of salt and ground black pepper
1 tsp coconut oil
quarter of an avocado
half a lemon, cut in two
1 tsp cilantro, chopped
salt and ground black pepper, to season
⅓ cup smoked salmon
2 cherry tomatoes, chopped
handful of arugula

1. Put the egg, herbs, beet, salt, and pepper into a blender. Mix well until everything is combined and the mixture is pink.

2. Heat a skillet over low heat and add the oil. Once the oil is melted, add the egg mixture and rotate the pan to let it all spread out thinly.

3. Leave to cook for approximately 3 minutes. Then flip the wrap on to the other side and cook for another few minutes, until it is firm.

4. In a bowl, mash the avocado, squeeze in the juice from one of the two wedges of lemon, and add some chopped cilantro (or any other herb you like). Season with salt and pepper.

5. Once the wrap is cooked, spread on the mashed avocado, add the smoked salmon, and sprinkle the arugula and tomato on top. Squeeze over the juice from the remaining lemon wedge and season with more pepper. Roll it up firmly and enjoy.

Top Tip Keep them fresh in the fridge by placing a piece of parchment paper in-between each wrap.

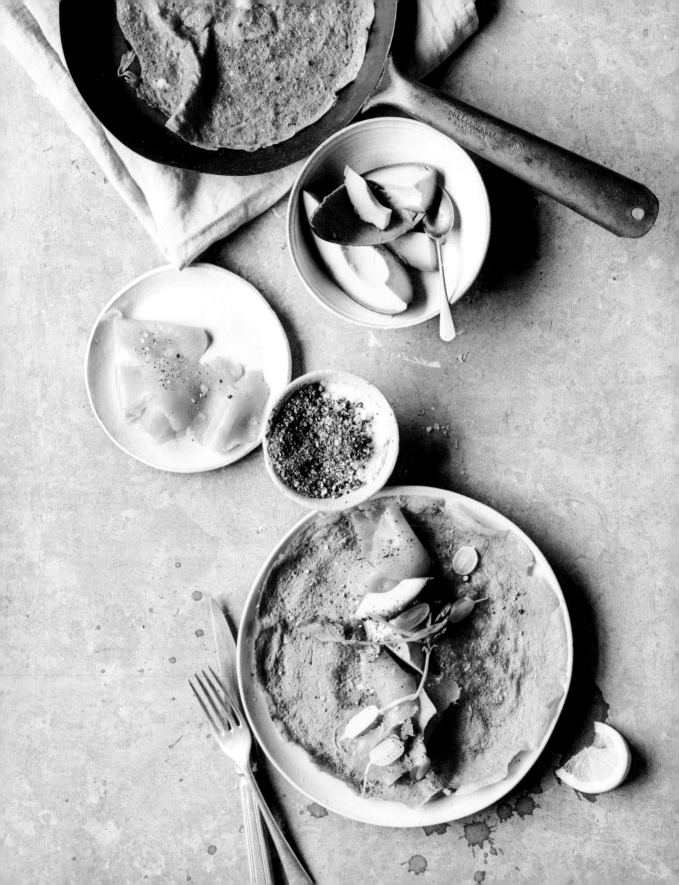

THE EGG BOWL

This is the best possible start you can have to the day. If you want to be kind to yourself, it's the ideal place to begin. This is such a heart-warming comfort food and one of the few dishes where the taste matches its wonderful health benefits. It's one of those dishes that never fails you—and it can easily be served at any time of the day.

serves 2

for the lemon tahini dressing
3 tbsp tahini
juice of 1 lemon
handful of cashews
handful of fresh parsley
salt and ground black pepper, to taste
½ cup water
drizzle of olive oil

for the bowl
3 tsp coconut oil
half a red onion, chopped
handful of pistachios, chopped
2 garlic cloves, crushed
1 cup buckwheat groats (cooked in stock, according to package instructions)
handful of fresh parsley, chopped, plus an extra sprig, to garnish
1 avocado, mashed, plus a few slices to garnish
juice of half a lemon
1 tsp chili flakes
2 handfuls of fresh spinach
2 organic, free-range eggs
2 tbsp sauerkraut (optional)

1. Put all the dressing ingredients in a blender and blend it up. Add more water until you get the perfect consistency. Season to taste.

2. Heat 1 teaspoon of the coconut oil in a skillet. Add the onion, pistachios, and half the garlic and season. Leave to sauté until soft and cooked through. Add the cooked buckwheat and mix everything together. Season to taste and add in the parsley.

3. Mix the avocado with the lemon juice and chili flakes. Season to taste.

4. In a skillet, heat another teaspoon of coconut oil and add the remaining garlic and then the spinach. Leave it to wilt.

5. Meanwhile, heat another skillet, add the remaining teaspoon of coconut oil, and fry the eggs.

6. Serve the buckwheat equally into two bowls, followed by the mashed avocado, wilted spinach, and a tablespoon of sauerkraut (if using).

7. Place a fried egg on the top of each bowl and drizzle with dressing and a sprig of parsley. Serve with the extra avocado slices.

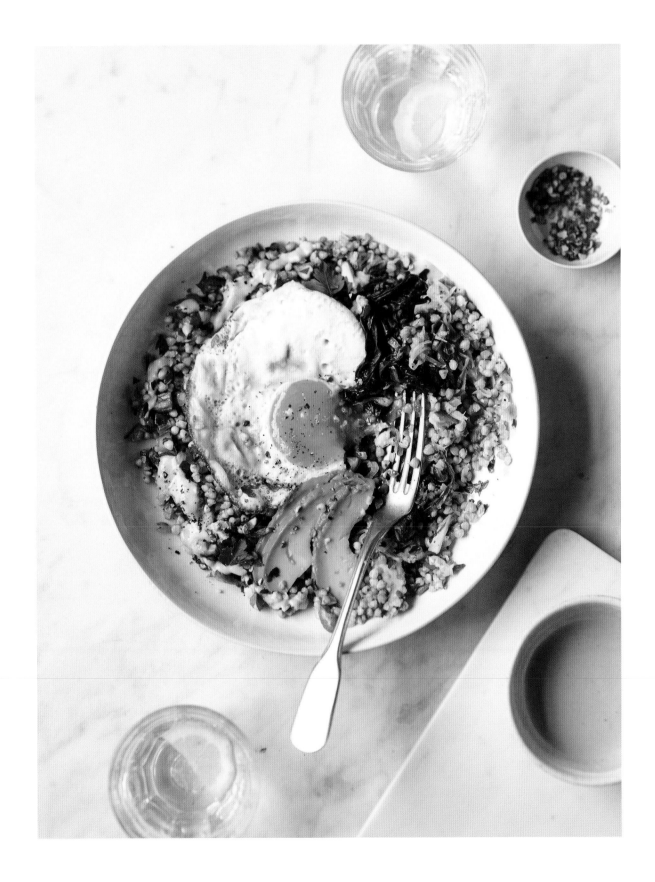

AVOCADO, TOMATO, AND CHILE SALSA WITH QUINOA BREAD

I love smashed avocado. I also love salsa. So I decided to mix them together! This salsa makes the perfect addition to ... literally everything. Have it with eggs, smother it on toast, or add it to your chicken or fish dish. If you aren't a fan of spice, then lower the amount of chile.

serves 4

3 avocados, peeled, pitted, and diced
half a red chile, seeded and finely chopped
¾-inch piece of fresh ginger root, finely grated
juice of 1 lime
½ tsp grated lime zest
1 scallion, finely chopped
pinch of Himalayan pink salt
small handful of fresh mint, chopped
small handful of cilantro, chopped
¾ cup cherry tomatoes, quartered

for the bread

½ cup uncooked quinoa, cooked with a pinch of salt, drained and cooled
½ cup flaxseeds
1 cup sunflower seeds, soaked for about 1 hour
1 cup pumpkin seeds
2 tbsp chia seeds
4 tbsp psyllium husks
1 tsp Himalayan pink salt
3 tbsp coconut oil, melted
1½ cups lukewarm water
1 tbsp maple syrup or honey

1. Start by making the bread. In a bowl, combine the quinoa along with the dry ingredients.

2. In a separate bowl, mix the coconut oil with the water and maple syrup or honey.

3. Combine the wet ingredients with the dry and stir until the mixture starts to thicken.

4. Line a 1-pound loaf pan with parchment paper, pour in the mixture, and allow to set for at least an hour or overnight.

5. Preheat the oven to 350°F.

6. Bake in the preheated oven for 45 minutes or until browned and pulling away from the parchment paper. Remove from the oven, allow to cool slightly, and remove from the pan and parchment paper, then return to the oven for up to 15 minutes to brown the outside.

7. To make the avocado salsa, simply mash the avocados in a mixing bowl, add in all of the remaining ingredients, and mix really well. Season to taste.

8. Slice the bread and toast it under the broiler. Spread on the salsa and enjoy. If you want to get all extravagant, then serve with a poached egg or two.

HEALTHY BREAKFAST HASH

This is a really filling breakfast that is a great vehicle for any leftover cooked or raw vegetables. If using potatoes, cook them from room temperature and give them a good five-minute head start on your other ingredients in the pan, as they take the longest to cook. Put a lid on the pan while cooking the potatoes to help speed things up. At the end, when cracking in the eggs, make sure the pan is off the heat so the bottom of the eggs don't burn; eggs are always best cooked low and slow.

serves 2
1 potato, diced into small cubes
1 sweet potato, diced into small cubes
1 tbsp coconut oil
1 red bell pepper, finely diced
2 scallions, chopped
handful of spinach or kale, chopped
¼ tsp salt
¼ tsp ground black pepper
2 organic, free-range eggs
pinch of chili flakes (optional)
fresh parsley or cilantro, to serve

1. Put the potatoes into a saucepan filled with boiling water and leave to cook for approximately 10 minutes, until cooked through, then drain.

2. Heat the oil in a medium-size skillet.

3. Throw the potatoes in and put the lid on. Every few minutes, give the potatoes a toss to make sure they are browning but not burning; having the lid on cooks them faster because they are searing and steaming at the same time.

4. After about 5 minutes of cooking time, turn down the heat and throw in the bell pepper, spinach, and scallions.

5. Add the salt and ground black pepper and cook for another minute.

6. Take the pan off the heat, make room in the pan and crack in the eggs. Season the eggs with a pinch of chili flakes and salt and pepper, if you like.

7. Put the pan back over medium to low heat and put the lid on.

8. Cook the eggs for about 2 minutes, or more if you like them well done.

9. Serve up the hash onto plates and put the eggs on top. Sprinkle with your freshly chopped herb of choice and enjoy a satisfying breakfast.

BRUNCHY BAKED EGGS

This is the perfect dish for a weekend brunch—it tastes delicious and looks impressive. Bear in mind that it's nearly impossible to get all the eggs baked to the same level—the ones in the middle will be runny and the ones at the edge crispy.

serves 4

10 oz/4 packed cups fresh spinach
1 tbsp olive oil or butter
1 small white onion, finely diced
2 garlic cloves, crushed
2 cups chopped mushrooms
3 tbsp light cream
pinch of freshly grated nutmeg (a little goes
   a long way)
¼ tsp salt
¼ tsp ground black pepper
4 organic, free-range eggs
1 tbsp grated Parmesan or a sprinkling
   of feta cheese (optional)

1. Preheat the oven to 350°F.

2. Cook the spinach in a small pan of boiling water until just wilted. This should take only 2 minutes.

3. Drain the spinach, and once cool, squeeze the liquid out of it with your hands and roughly chop it up.

4. Heat the oil or butter over medium heat in an ovenproof skillet and sauté the onion for 3 minutes, until softened.

5. Add the garlic and cook for another minute.

6. Add the mushrooms and stir, allowing the mix to cook for another 3 minutes.

7. Add in your drained, chopped spinach, the cream, nutmeg, salt, and pepper. Stir everything together and let the flavors distribute evenly while bringing to a simmer for 1–2 minutes.

8. Take the pan off the heat and make 4 indentations in the mixture with the back of a large spoon.

9. Crack an egg into each dent, sprinkle lightly with salt and pepper, and put the pan in the oven. Leave it to cook for about 6 minutes and check it.

10. You want the whites to have set but the yolks to be runny. If the egg whites still look raw, give it another 2 minutes in the oven.

11. Take the dish out and sprinkle the cheese on top, if desired. Serve up immediately with buttered slices of your favorite toast, or enjoy on its own!

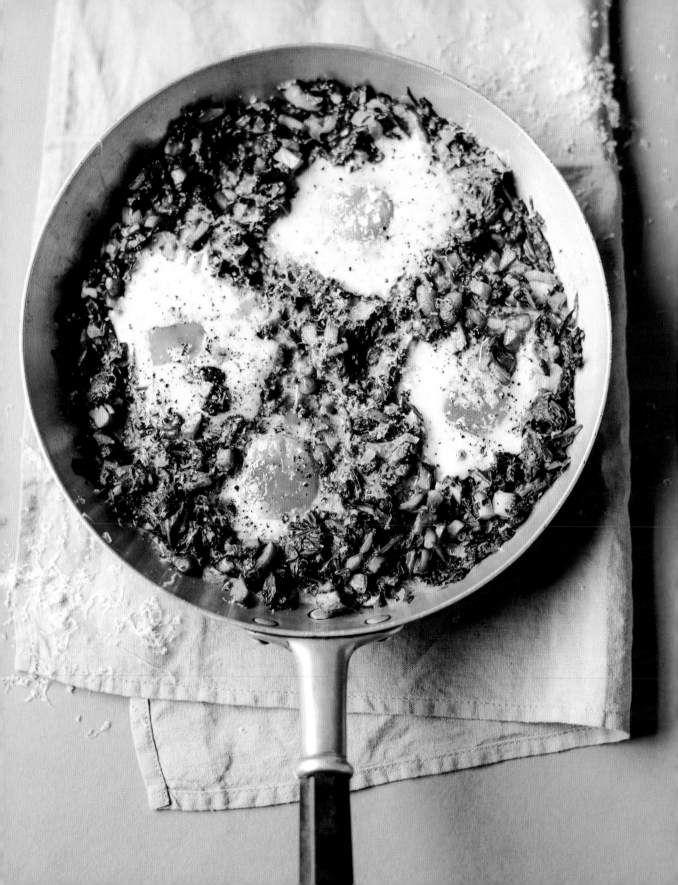

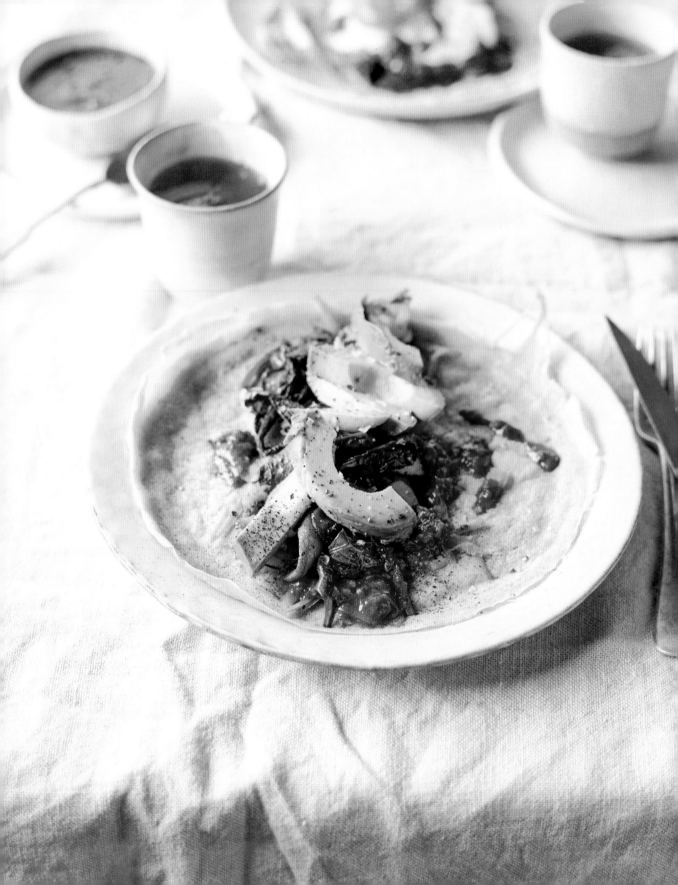

BUCKWHEAT, EGG, CARROT, AND MUSHROOM CRÊPES

Breakfast crêpe recipes are generally laden with sugary sweet fillings; this savory crêpe is something I discovered in Australia, and it's perfect for brunch or even lunch. I love the addition of the crunchy sweet carrots and thyme in this dish. Buckwheat crêpes are beautifully light so it is important to keep the batter in the fridge because it keeps them fluffy and delicious.

serves 4

2¾ cups buckwheat flour
2 tsp Himalayan pink salt
3¼ cups filtered water
5 organic, free-range eggs
3 carrots
5 large portobello mushrooms
2 tbsp coconut oil
1 tbsp fresh thyme leaves
10 oz/4 packed cups fresh spinach
salt and ground black pepper, to season
1 tsp black sesame seeds, to garnish

1. Combine the flour and salt and gradually add the water, a little at a time, stirring after each addition. Add one egg and incorporate into the mixture. Put the batter in the fridge for 1–2 hours, because this will make the crêpes nice and fluffy.

2. While the batter is in the fridge, coarsely grate the carrot and finely slice the mushrooms. Heat 1 tablespoon of the coconut oil in a skillet and lightly fry the mushrooms with the fresh thyme. After 2 minutes, stir in the spinach and cook until the spinach is wilted. This should take 5 minutes. Remove from the heat and set aside.

3. Heat the remaining coconut oil in a nonstick skillet and ladle in the crêpe mixture, swirling it around the pan to create a nice thin layer. Fry until the edges start to crisp and then flip over and cook on the other side. Repeat this process for all the crêpes and set aside. Meanwhile, fry the remaining eggs in a separate pan.

4. Place a crêpe on a plate and sprinkle a quarter of the grated carrot, mushroom and spinach mixture down the middle. Season, then top with a fried egg and fold over. Garnish with black sesame seeds.

Top Tip This dish is delicious with a spoonful of Homemade Harissa (page 185).

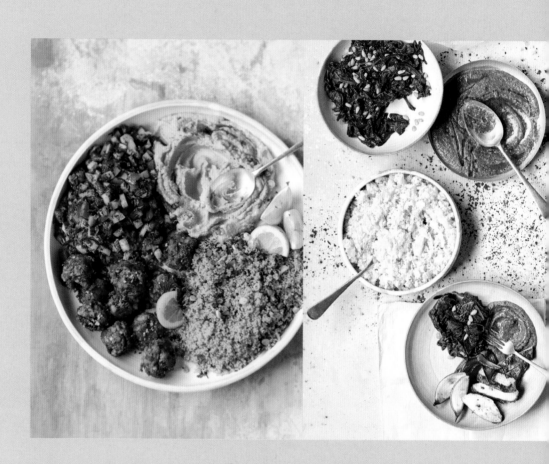

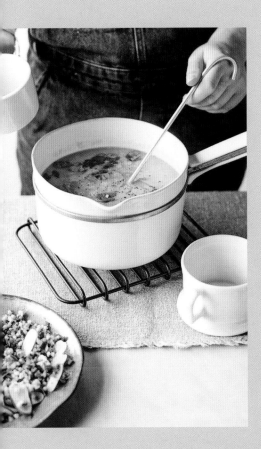

LUNCH

Immune bowl

Omega-3 Bowl

Happy Bowl

Middle Eastern Bowl

Fish Stick Sandwich

Miso Shrimp and Eggplant Salad

Chickpea Dosa Wrap

Kabbouleh

Bodyism Frittata

Alkalizing Supergreen Soup

Turmeric, Sweet Potato, Ginger, and Coconut Soup

BOWLS

Bowls are the foodie way forward. The amazing thing about them is that you can mix and match each part to tailor-make your very own nutrient-rich lunch. You can make a large amount of each component and just spoon it into a container each day, or you can make the bowls look beautiful and invite a load of friends round to enjoy them together. Choose your base and add the protein, veggies, and a spoon of dip on top. Each bowl serves 4.

IMMUNE BOWL

for the base (brown rice)
¾ cup brown rice
2 cups bone broth (see Miracle Bone Broth recipe on page 159), or if you don't have bone broth, use stock instead
2 cups water
salt and ground black pepper, to season
1 tbsp olive oil
1 onion, chopped
1 garlic clove, crushed

1. Wash the brown rice in a strainer before placing it in a large saucepan. Add the broth and water and place over high heat to bring to a boil. Once it's boiling, lower the heat. Season with salt and pepper. Leave to cook for 15–20 minutes, until the rice is cooked through.

2. In a skillet, add the olive oil and place over low heat. Add the onion and garlic and leave to sauté for approximately 5 minutes, until the onion has softened.

3. Pour the onion and garlic into the saucepan and mix through.

for the protein (turkey meatballs)
2¼ cups ground turkey
2 carrots, grated
1 zucchini, grated
2 tbsp tomato paste
2 tbsp mixed Italian seasoning
1 onion
salt and ground black pepper, to season
1 organic, free-range egg
1 tbsp coconut oil

1. Place the ground turkey in a mixing bowl. Stir in the carrots, zucchini, tomato paste, Italian seasoning, and the onion. Season with salt and pepper and mix. Stir in the egg.

2. Wet your hands and roll a tablespoon of the mixture into a ball and place on a baking tray. Continue to do this until all the mixture is used up—it should be enough for 12 balls.

3. Heat a large skillet over medium heat and add the oil. Once it is melted, cook the meatballs for 5–6 minutes, or until cooked through and nicely browned on the outside. You'll probably have to repeat the process for a second batch, unless you have a very large pan.

for the veggies (charred broccoli and chile)

2 heads of broccoli (about 1 lb 2 oz),
　cut into florets
½ cup olive oil
coarse sea salt and freshly ground black
　pepper
4 garlic cloves, thinly sliced
1 red chile, seeded and thinly sliced
½ cup slivered almonds, toasted

1. Fill a large saucepan with water and bring to a boil. Throw in the broccoli and blanch for 2 minutes. Drain the broccoli and transfer it to a bowl full of ice-cold water. Drain and use paper towels to dry completely. In a mixing bowl; toss the broccoli with 3 tablespoons of the oil and a generous pinch of salt and pepper.

2. Place a grill pan over high heat until it is extremely hot (approximately 3 minutes). Broil the broccoli in several batches, turning them around as they broil so they get char marks all over. Transfer to a heatproof bowl and continue with another batch.

3. While broiling the broccoli, place the remaining oil in a small saucepan with the garlic and chile. Cook them over medium heat until the garlic just begins to turn golden brown. Be careful not to let the garlic and chile burn. Pour the oil mixture over the hot broccoli and mix together well. Taste and adjust the seasoning.

4. Garnish the broccoli with the toasted almonds before serving.

for the dip (ratatouille)

1 tbsp rapeseed/canola oil
1 onion, chopped
2 garlic cloves, crushed
salt and ground black pepper, to season
2 x 14-oz cans organic chopped tomatoes
1 tbsp dried oregano
1 tbsp red wine vinegar
1 tbsp tomato paste
2 bell peppers, seeded and chopped

1. Heat the oil in a large saucepan. Add the onion and garlic and leave to sauté over low heat for 5 minutes, until the onion softens. Season with salt and pepper.

2. Pour in the tomatoes, oregano, vinegar, tomato paste, and bell peppers and stir well. Cook over low heat for 15–20 minutes.

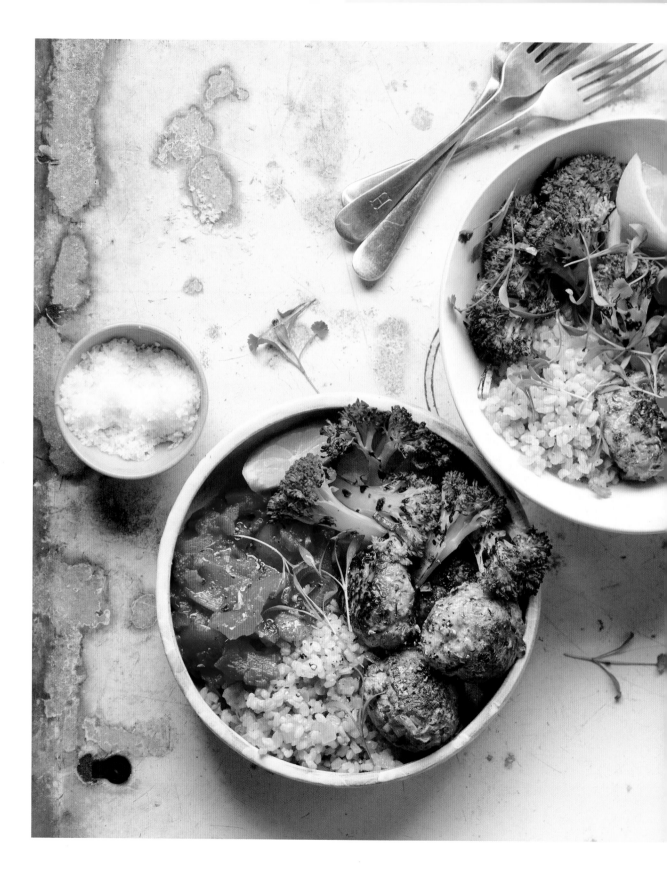

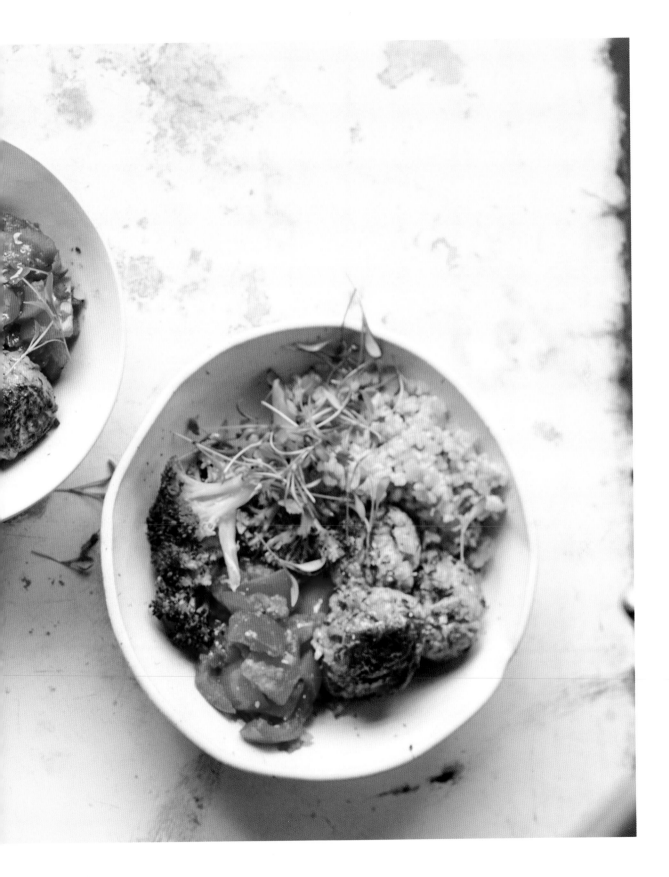

OMEGA-3 BOWL

for the base (kelp noodles)
12 oz/3 cups kelp noodles
2 tbsp tamari
4 tbsp sesame oil
½ cup cashews, toasted and chopped

1. Rinse the kelp noodles in warm water for about 10 minutes. This will soften and separate them. Drain the noodles and, using kitchen scissors, cut them into small pieces.

2. Mix the kelp noodles with the tamari and sesame oil. Stir in the toasted cashews.

---

for the protein (miso-glazed salmon)
1 tbsp miso paste
¾-inch piece of fresh ginger root, grated
4 tbsp coconut milk
2 tbsp tamari
3 scallions, finely chopped
juice of 1 lime
4 organic salmon fillets (approximately 9 oz each)

1. Preheat the oven to 350°F.

2. Whisk the miso paste, ginger, coconut milk, tamari, scallions, and lime together to make the marinade and season to taste.

3. Place the salmon fillets in a deep baking dish and pour the marinade into the dish. Cover with foil. Leave to marinate for a minimum of 2 hours (or overnight).

4. Place in the oven for 12–15 minutes, until cooked. Once cool, slice into flakes.

---

for the veggies (bok choy and chile)
1 tbsp sesame oil
1 tbsp coconut oil
1 large garlic clove, crushed
half a red chile, seeded and finely chopped
1 bok choy
1 tbsp tamari

1. Place a lidded wok over medium heat and add the oils. Once melted, add the garlic and chile and lower the heat. Leave to sauté for 2–3 minutes.

2. Add the bok choy and toss until coated with the garlic and chile mixture. Cover with the lid and leave to cook for 5 minutes.

3. Take the wok off the heat. Pour over the tamari and toss well.

for the dip (edamame and ginger dip)
1½ cups frozen shelled edamame
¼ cup water
2 tbsp tamari
2 tsp fresh ginger root, minced
1 tbsp rice vinegar
1 tbsp tahini
1 garlic clove, chopped
pinch of salt

1. Cook the edamame as instructed on the package.

2. Put all the ingredients into a blender and blend until smooth.

3. Season to taste.

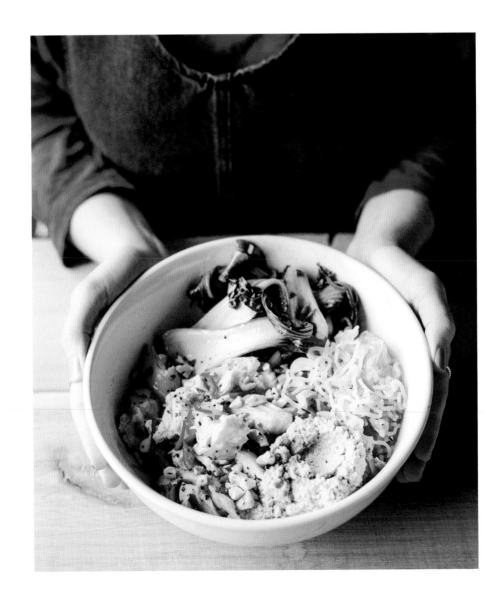

HAPPY BOWL

for the base (cauliflower rice)
2 cauliflowers, florets only
1 tsp coconut oil
1 onion, finely chopped
2 garlic cloves, crushed
salt and ground black pepper, to season

1. To make the cauliflower rice, pulse the cauliflower in the bowl of a food processor until it resembles rice (about 2–3 minutes); set aside.

2. Heat a large skillet over low heat and add the oil. Add the onion and garlic and leave to sauté for 5 minutes, until the onion is soft.

3. Mix in the cauliflower rice.

4. Season to taste.

---

for the protein (harissa chicken)
4 organic chicken breasts (approximately 5¼ oz each)
4 tbsp Homemade Harissa (page 185), or opt for a good-quality store-bought one with no added sugar
1 tbsp coconut oil
2 red onions, quartered

1. Coat the chicken with harissa.

2. Heat a large grill pan over medium heat. Once hot, add the coconut oil. When it has melted, add the chicken and cook on each side for 3–4 minutes, until lightly charred and cooked through.

3. Add the onions after the chicken has been cooking for 4 minutes and leave to sauté for 5 minutes until the onion is soft. Remove from the heat.

---

for the veggies (wilted spinach, garlic, and pine nuts)
1¾ lbs/11 packed cups fresh spinach
3 tbsp rapeseed/canola oil
2 garlic cloves, finely chopped
3 tbsp pine nuts

1. Wash the spinach and place into a large saucepan. Pour over a little boiling water and cover for 2–3 minutes while the spinach wilts.

2. Drain the spinach in a colander.

3. In a skillet, heat the oil and add the garlic and pine nuts. Fry until golden (approximately 3 minutes).

4. Stir in the spinach and season to taste.

for the dip (azuki bean mash):
1 tsp coconut oil
1 onion, finely chopped
1 garlic clove, crushed
2 tsp ground cumin
1 tsp ground coriander
salt and ground black pepper, to season
1 x 14-oz can organic azuki beans, drained
⅓ cup water

1. Heat a skillet and add the oil. Once melted, add the onion and garlic and sauté for 5 minutes, until the onion has softened.

2. Add the cumin and coriander and mix well. Season with salt and pepper.

3. Pour the drained beans and the water into a blender. Pour in the onion and garlic mixture.

4. Blend until all the ingredients are well combined.

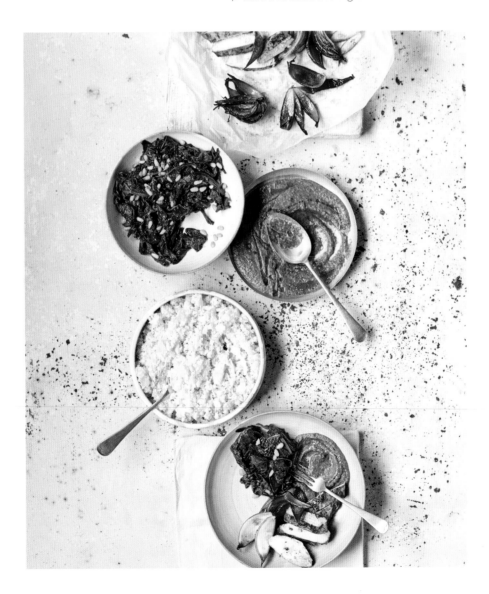

MIDDLE EASTERN BOWL

for the base (quinoa)

1 cup uncooked quinoa
2 tsp ground turmeric
juice of 1 lemon
2 tbsp tamari
⅓ cup fresh parsley, finely chopped
⅓ cup cilantro, finely chopped
2 scallions, finely chopped

1. Rinse the quinoa in water to remove its bitter flavor. Tip into a large saucepan and add salted water to a volume that is approximately double that of the quinoa. Add the turmeric, lemon juice, and tamari. Place on a boil for 15 minutes, until the quinoa is cooked but still retains a slight bite.

2. Fluff it up with a fork and then mix in the parsley, cilantro, and scallions. Season to taste.

for the protein (beet falafel)

¾ cup uncooked chickpeas (garbanzo beans)
1 garlic clove, crushed
1 tsp paprika
5¼ oz/¾ cup cooked beet, chopped
zest of 1 lemon
1 tbsp cilantro, finely chopped
1 tbsp buckwheat flour
½ tsp baking soda

1. Soak the chickpeas in water and a pinch of salt overnight. In the morning, drain and dry thoroughly.

2. Preheat the oven to 350°F and line a baking sheet with parchment paper.

3. Heat the oil in a skillet and add the garlic and paprika. Leave to sauté for 2–3 minutes.

4. Pour the chickpeas, beet, garlic mixture, lemon, and cilantro into a food processor and blend it up. Add the flour and baking soda and blend again.

5. Using damp hands, roll the mixture into even-size balls and place on the baking sheet. Brush lightly with oil and bake for 20–25 minutes, until crisp and warm.

for the veggies (Israeli salad)

1 cucumber, diced
4 plum tomatoes, seeded and finely
   chopped
1 red bell pepper, finely chopped
⅔ cup fresh parsley, chopped
⅔ cup fresh mint, chopped
juice of 1 lemon
¼ cup olive oil
salt and ground black pepper, to season

1. In a bowl, mix the cucumber, tomatoes, bell pepper, parsley, and mint.

2. Add the lemon juice and oil and mix well. Season to taste.

for the dip (butternut squash hummus)
7 oz/1½ cups butternut squash, peeled and
    chopped into cubes
2 garlic cloves, peeled
1 tbsp coconut oil, melted
juice of 1 lemon
1 x 14-oz can chickpeas (garbanzo beans),
    drained and rinsed
2 tbsp tahini
4 tbsp olive oil
2 tbsp cilantro, chopped
salt and ground black pepper, to season

1. Preheat the oven to 350°F and line a baking sheet
   with parchment paper.

2. Place the squash and garlic cloves on the sheet and
   drizzle with coconut oil. Place in the preheated oven
   for 20 minutes, until cooked through. Leave to cool.

3. Put the squash into a food processor. Add all the
   other ingredients apart from one of the garlic cloves
   and mix until well combined. Season to taste.

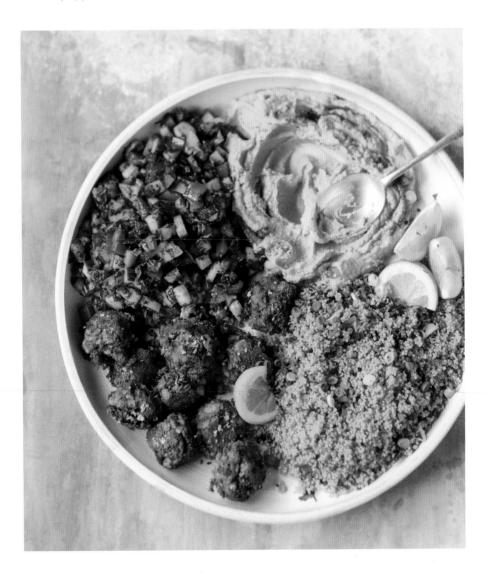

FISH STICK SANDWICH

This is the Bodyism take on a fish-stick sandwich for when you want some pure comfort food—your body will thank you for it.

serves 2
10 oz/4 packed cups fresh spinach
4 slices organic sourdough bread
2 handfuls of sliced iceberg lettuce
sweet potato fries, to serve
lemon wedges, to serve

for the tartare sauce
3 tbsp organic Greek yogurt
½ tsp horseradish
1 tbsp chopped fresh chives
salt and ground black pepper, to season

for the smashed avocado
1 avocado
juice of half a lemon
pinch of chili flakes
salt and ground black pepper, to season

for the fish sticks
¾ cup buckwheat flour
¾ cup brown rice flour
1 cup ground almonds
1 tsp garlic powder
1 tsp dried parsley
zest of 1 lemon
salt and ground black pepper, to season
3 organic, free-range eggs
7 oz organic (or locally sourced), skinless
   haddock loin (or any other line-caught
   white fish)
2 tsp rapeseed/canola oil or olive oil

1. Heat the broiler to medium temperature.

2. Mix the tartare sauce ingredients together and leave in the fridge while you make everything else.

3. Make the smashed avocado by mashing the avocado add adding the lemon juice, chili flakes, and salt and pepper. Mix well.

4. For the fish fingers, mix the buckwheat flour, rice flour, ground almonds, garlic powder, parsley, lemon zest, and salt and pepper in a bowl and mix well.

5. In a separate bowl, crack the eggs and whisk.

6. Slice the haddock into 4 chunky sticks.

7. Dip one piece of fish at a time into the egg and then the flour mix. To make them extra crunchy, repeat this step.

8. Put a skillet over medium heat and add a splash of oil. When the pan is hot, add the sticks (you might need to do this in batches) and fry for approximately 3 minutes each side, or until they are cooked through, golden, and crispy. Remove to a double layer of paper towels to drain while you fry the next batch (add more oil if needed).

9. Broil the bread while the fish is cooking.

10. Spread the smashed avocado on 2 slices of the toasted bread. Put a handful of iceberg lettuce on top of each, followed by two fish sticks. Finish each sandwich with the remaining toast, spread with the tartare sauce. Serve on a plate with sweet potato fries and lemon wedges.

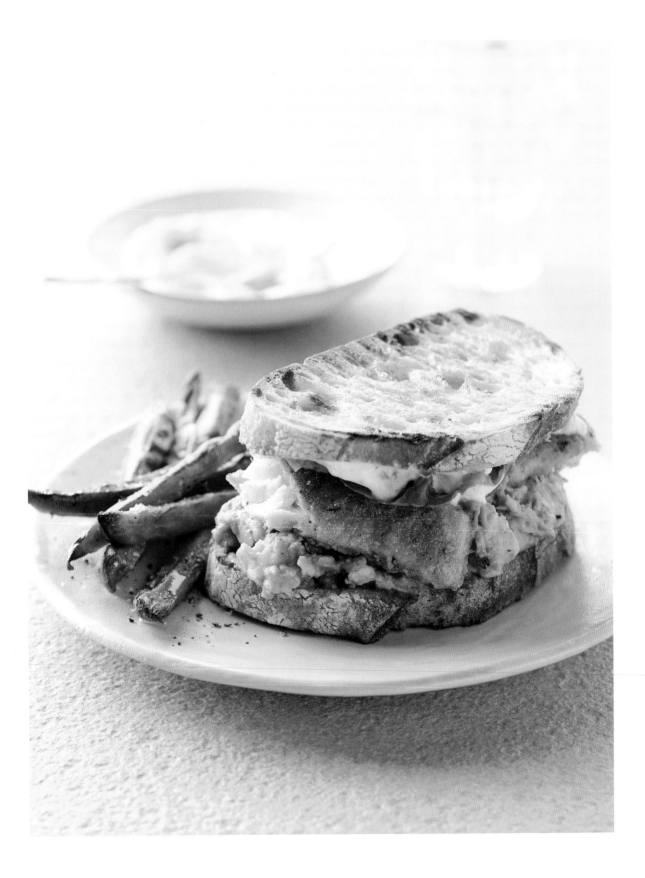

MISO SHRIMP AND EGGPLANT SALAD

I love this Asian-inspired salad; it's the perfect combination of sweet (from the coconut) and salt (from the tamari). Most dressings are packed with sugar, so make sure you read the bottle if you opt for a store-bought one. Eggplants are such great additions to salads because they are quite filling, they absorb the dressing really well, and are really easy to cook. If you don't want shrimp, then add any other protein you fancy—chicken, salmon, turkey, or some chickpeas.

serves 4

14 oz buckwheat soba noodles
1 tbsp coconut oil
2 eggplants, diced
half a red chile, seeded and finely chopped
12 large raw tiger shrimp
2 tbsp coconut milk
⅓ cup brown miso paste
2 tbsp sesame oil
3 tbsp tamari
1½-inch piece of fresh ginger root, grated
1 tbsp rice wine vinegar
4 scallions, finely chopped
⅔ cup coconut flakes, toasted
cilantro leaves, to serve

1. Bring a pan of water to a boil and cook the noodles following the package instructions.

2. Heat the coconut oil in a large skillet until melted. Cook the eggplants and chile over medium heat for 8–10 minutes, until softened.

3. In the last few minutes of cooking the eggplants, throw in the shrimp and leave them to turn opaque—it should take about 3 minutes.

4. Mix together the coconut milk, miso, sesame oil, tamari, ginger, and vinegar.

5. Drain the noodles and add to the pan of shrimp and eggplants. Pour over the dressing and serve with a scattering of scallions, toasted coconut flakes, and cilantro leaves.

CHICKPEA DOSA WRAP

I love a wrap, and I throw anything I can find into it! This chickpea wrap is one of my absolute favorites because it is so easy to make. Often, I make them in bulk and then just grab one from the fridge when I'm in a rush. Experiment with adding different dried spices and herbs into the batter.

serves 4

2¼ cups chickpea/gram flour
salt and ground black pepper, to season
1⅔ cups water
1 tbsp coconut oil
1 garlic clove, crushed
1 shallot, finely chopped
half a red bell pepper, finely chopped
1 tbsp rapeseed/canola oil

for the filling

2 tbsp Butternut Squash Hummus
  (page 129)
half an avocado, sliced
1 plum tomato, sliced
slices of Harissa Chicken (page 126),
  or any other fillings you fancy

1. Put the flour in a mixing bowl and season with salt and pepper. Make a well in the center of the flour and pour in the water slowly, while whisking, until well combined. Set the batter aside for at least half an hour.

2. Heat an 8-inch skillet and add the coconut oil. Add the garlic, shallot, and red pepper. Sauté over low heat for 5 minutes, until the shallot has softened. Take off the heat and leave to cool.

3. Pour the shallot, garlic, and red pepper into the flour mixture and stir well.

4. Heat a small skillet and add the rapeseed oil. Once the pan is very hot and the oil has spread across the pan, pour in a small ladle of the batter. Spread the mixture across the base of the pan and leave to cook for approximately 3 minutes. Using a spatula, flip the dosa over and leave to cook on the other side. Remove from the pan and repeat until all the batter is used up.

5. Spread the hummus on each wrap and pile up with fillings. Wrap up and enjoy!

KABBOULEH

This is a delicious lunch-box treat or the perfect accompaniment to any protein. Feel free to mix up your grains and use what you have on hand—simply sauté any leftover grains in a little olive oil rather than cooking them fresh. If you're gluten-intolerant, avoid couscous and bulgur wheat, and use quinoa or brown rice instead. Use this salad as a vehicle for leftover vegetables—the choice is yours!

serves 4

3 tbsp extra virgin olive oil
¼ tsp ground cumin
½ tsp sumac
juice of 1 lemon
¼ tsp salt
¼ tsp ground black pepper
3 handfuls of kale (stalks discarded), finely chopped
half a small cucumber, seeds scooped out, finely chopped
1 scallion, finely chopped
8 small tomatoes, chopped into quarters
handful of fresh parsley, finely chopped
½ cup cooked and cooled quinoa, brown rice or bulgur wheat (or any leftover cooked grains you have)

1. First, make the dressing; it will taste better the longer it sits. Whisk together the olive oil, cumin, sumac, lemon juice, salt, and pepper and set aside.

2. Put the kale, cucumber, scallion, and tomatoes into a serving bowl and stir in the parsley.

3. Pour over half the dressing and mix it through; this step will tenderize the kale and distribute great flavor through the salad.

4. Add in your cooled grains and the rest of your dressing, stirring everything together. It's important to make sure the grains have cooled down completely before adding them, so they don't wilt the salad—you want fresh, crisp bites, not soggy ones.

5. Taste the salad for seasoning and add more salt or another squeeze of lemon if needed. Make it your own and add as much or as little of the seasonings as you like! Dig in and enjoy every bite.

Top Tip If you like heat, feel free to add in a little fresh or dried chile, or some finely chopped garlic.

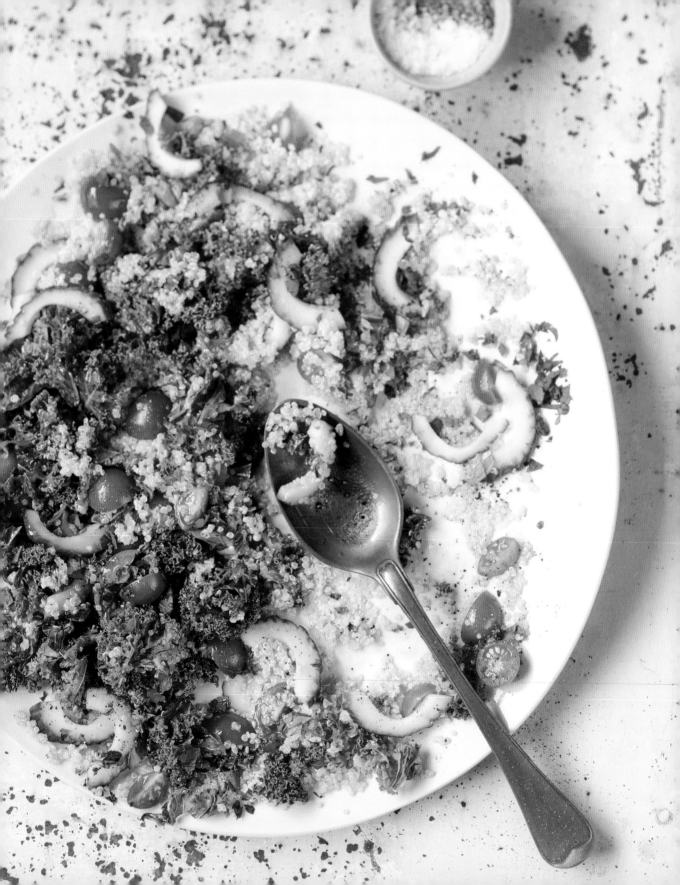

BODYISM FRITTATA

This is such a delicious way to use up any leftover vegetables in the fridge. Use this recipe as your guide and feel free to swap any vegetables or herbs with what you have available.

serves 4
1 tbsp coconut oil
2 garlic cloves, crushed
3 zucchini, sliced into discs
1 leek, sliced
4 mushrooms, sliced
8 organic, free-range eggs
salt and ground black pepper, to season
1 tbsp dried mixed herbs
handful of vegetables (leftover roasted
    squash, parsnips, red bell pepper, or peas
    from the freezer)
handful of organic cheddar/sharp cheese,
    grated (optional)

1. Heat the broiler to high.

2. Heat a large ovenproof skillet on the stovetop and add the coconut oil. Once melted, add the garlic, zucchini, leek, and mushrooms. Leave to sauté for 5–8 minutes, until the leek and zucchini are soft. Let cool.

3. Beat the eggs in a bowl and season well. Add the mixed herbs and your chosen vegetables.

4. Pour the egg mixture into the skillet with the zucchini and cook over low heat for 8–10 minutes.

5. If you are adding cheese, sprinkle on top and place the pan under the broiler for 3–5 minutes, until set.

6. Cut into thick wedges and serve. This also makes a delicious breakfast—so keep the leftovers and enjoy the next day.

ALKALIZING SUPERGREEN SOUP

This soup is filled with alkalizing greens and nourishing broth. It is one of those dishes that will make you feel a little bit smug because it is just so ridiculously good for you. The key with soups and stews is to build the flavor by seasoning as you go and to follow the initial steps properly. In this case, make sure you have sautéed the onions until translucent and given the garlic a minute or two to cook before adding the parsnip and broth. These initial steps will really bring a sweetness and depth of flavor to the soup. If you want a thicker soup, feel free to add extra parsnip.

This soup will keep in your fridge for up to three days. I like to eat half and freeze the rest for a rainy day.

serves 4, with leftovers

1 tbsp olive oil
1 large white onion, chopped
2 large garlic cloves, crushed
½ tsp salt
½ tsp freshly ground pepper
1 parsnip, peeled and diced into small cubes
4 cups chicken stock or vegetable stock (top up with hot water, if desired)
2 large handfuls of kale (stalks discarded)
4 large handfuls of fresh spinach
1 large handful of cavolo nero (stalks discarded)

1. Heat the olive oil in a large stockpot over medium heat. Sauté the onion until translucent, for about 2 minutes.

2. Add the garlic and half the salt and pepper and allow to cook for about 2 minutes. You don't want to add the stock while the garlic is raw.

3. Add in your diced parsnip and stir. Pour in 4 cups of whatever stock you have chosen (I prefer chicken stock) and top off with hot water, if desired.

4. Add the kale, spinach, and cavolo nero. Turn up the heat and allow the soup to come to a boil, then turn down to a low simmer.

5. Add the remaining salt and pepper and stir in. Let the soup simmer and the flavors develop for about 20 minutes.

6. Blend to a smooth consistency using a food processor or hand-held stick blender (be careful, please!) and simmer over low heat for another 30 minutes.

7. Taste and add more salt or pepper, or perhaps a dash of cream for richness, if desired.

8. Make the soup your own and enjoy!

TURMERIC, SWEET POTATO, GINGER, AND COCONUT SOUP

This is such a bright and beautiful soup. It's filled with nourishing ingredients to zap away those change-of-weather colds. I like making a big batch and freezing it for a simple supper. It's the perfect autumnal soup.

serves 5

1 tbsp coconut oil
2 red onions, diced
1 head of celery, diced
thumb of fresh ginger root, grated
3 medium-size sweet potatoes, peeled and
   cut into chunks
2 tsp ground turmeric
1 x 14-fl oz can organic coconut milk
juice of 1 lime
cilantro, to serve

1. Heat the coconut oil in a large, heavy saucepan until melted. Add the red onions and the celery and sauté for 5 minutes.

2. Add the grated ginger and sweet potato and simmer for a further 5 minutes. Cover with boiling water, so the pan is about two-thirds full.

3. Add the turmeric and simmer for 15 minutes, until the sweet potato is soft.

4. Turn off the heat, add the coconut milk, and blend with a hand-held stick blender or food processor.

5. Pour back into the saucepan and simmer, being careful not to bring to a boil.

6. Add the lime juice and season to taste. Pour into bowls and garnish with cilantro.

Top Tip The sweet potato can be substituted with squash to make a delicious bright and light soup.

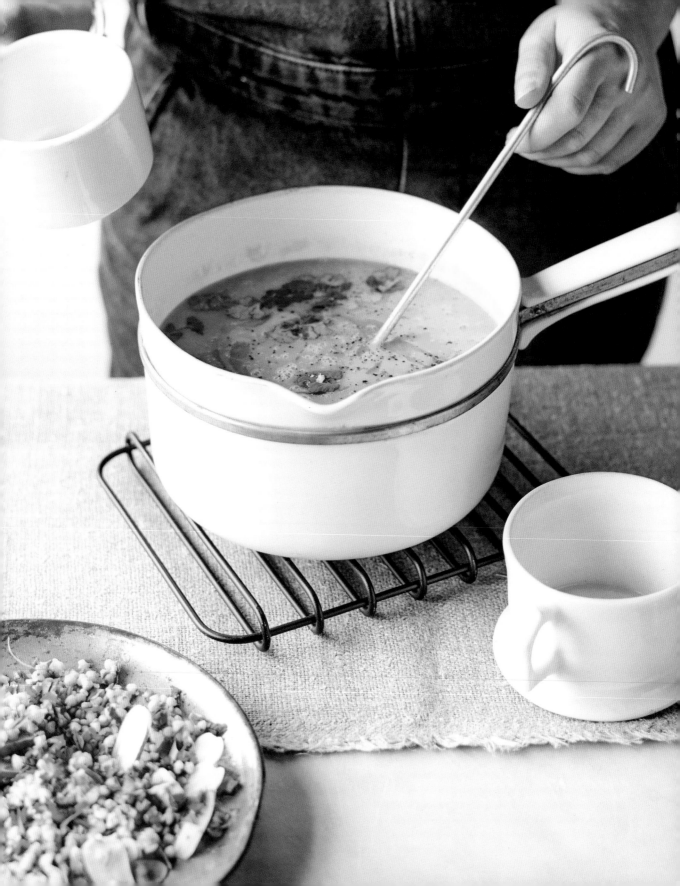

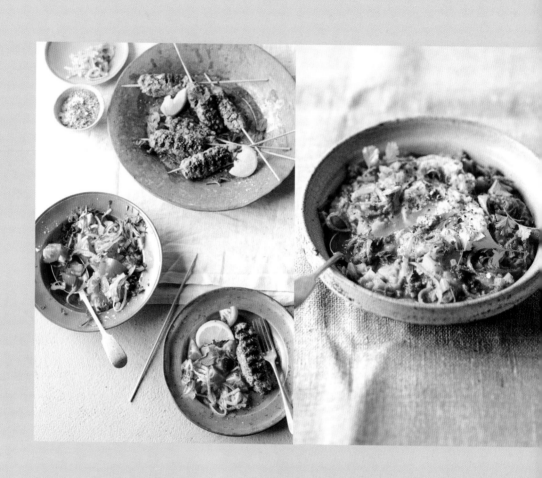

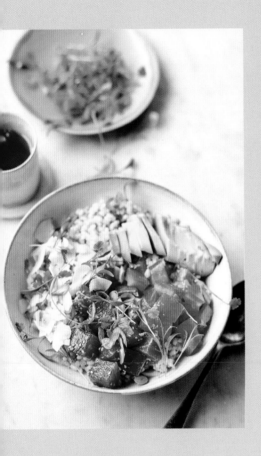

DINNER

Zucchini Lasagna

Ultimate Fish Pie

Dukkah-Crusted Salmon with Asian Brussels Sprout Salad

Turmeric Dal

Sticky Chicken Thighs

Lamb Koftas with Tomato and Onion Salad

Moroccan Tagine

Tuna Poké Bowl

Middle Eastern Meatballs

Sexy Stir-Fry

Slow-Cooked Irish Stew

Miracle Bone Broth

Poached Coconut Chicken and Cauli-Rice

Keralan Fish Curry

Perfect Roast Chicken

Chicken Schnitzel with Root Vegetable Mash

The Perfect Burger

Leftover Roast Chicken Pho

Shrimp Summer Rolls with Tamari Dipping Sauce

ZUCCHINI LASAGNA

This lasagna is a much healthier version than the traditional recipe, but that doesn't take away from its taste. The meat sauce is packed with flavor, and I like to leave it cooking away for hours, just to make it all the more intense. If you want, you can swap the zucchini with layers of thinly sliced squash or sweet potato, but I do like the zucchini best.

serves 4

1 tbsp coconut oil
1 onion, chopped
2 garlic cloves, finely chopped
1 tsp ground nutmeg
1 tsp ground cinnamon
1 tbsp dried oregano
handful of fresh basil, finely chopped
2 tbsp tomato paste
1 tsp Worcestershire sauce
1 lb 2 oz lean organic ground lamb
1 x 14-oz can chopped tomatoes
1 tbsp red wine vinegar
4 zucchini, sliced into ribbons with a peeler
1 cup sliced mushrooms
Parmesan cheese, grated

1. Preheat the oven to 400°F.

2. Heat the oil in a large skillet over medium heat and sauté the onion and garlic for approximately 5 minutes, until softened.

3. Add the nutmeg, cinnamon, oregano, basil, tomato paste, and Worcestershire sauce and mix well. Add the lamb and cook for 10 minutes, until brown.

4. Stir in the tomatoes and vinegar and simmer for 15–20 minutes.

5. In a large baking dish, spoon a layer of the mixture, topped with a layer of zucchini ribbons and then a layer of mushrooms. Repeat, finishing with a layer of zucchini ribbons.

6. Sprinkle the Parmesan over the top and bake for 15–20 minutes.

7. Serve with a fresh green salad.

ULTIMATE FISH PIE

Fish pie reminds me of after-school dinners. Full of flavor, protein, and vegetables, it's one of those home comforts, and this version is wonderful for you, too.

This is a dish that you can really play with and adapt to your own tastes. Use any firm white fish, from cod to pollock. Vary up the mash—try creamy potatoes, rutabaga or even cauliflower—it's entirely up to you. Get your mash started first, so the celery root can boil while you're preparing the pie.

serves 4
½ tsp butter
½ tsp olive oil
1 white onion, chopped
2 large garlic cloves, minced
2 carrots, peeled and chopped
1 leek, white part only, chopped
½ tsp salt
½ tsp ground black pepper
3 cups whole milk
1 bay leaf
1 tbsp arrowroot powder
14 oz cod, chopped into bite-size chunks
7 oz smoked haddock, chopped into
    bite-size chunks
6 oz shrimp
large handful of fresh parsley, including
    stalks, chopped

for the mash
2 small celery roots, peeled and cut
    into chunks
pinch of salt
¼ tsp ground black pepper
½ tbsp butter

1. Preheat the oven to 350°F.

2. To make the mash, add the celery root and salt to a pan of water and bring to a boil. Turn the heat down and simmer gently for 20 minutes. Drain and mash the celery root, adding the pepper and butter. Set aside.

3. Put the butter and olive oil together in a large skillet and melt over medium heat. Add the onion and sauté for 3 minutes, until softened.

4. Add the garlic and sauté for another 1–2 minutes, until you can smell its garlicky aroma. Add the carrots and leek and half the salt and pepper, and stir everything together.

5. Turn the heat down and pour in the milk, also adding the bay leaf. After 1–2 minutes, scoop a ladleful of the milk mixture into a cup and whisk in the arrowroot. This will thicken the sauce.

6. Add the whisked milk and arrowroot back into the pan and stir. Add the fish and shrimp. The fish will poach in the milk and impart a lovely smoky flavor into the dish.

7. Add another pinch of salt and pepper to the liquid and throw in all the parsley. Allow this mix to simmer for about 6 minutes, until the fish is cooked.

8. Transfer the mixture to a baking dish. Top with the mashed celery root and place in the preheated oven. Bake for 25 minutes until bubbling at the edges.

DUKKAH-CRUSTED SALMON WITH ASIAN BRUSSELS SPROUT SALAD

This is another easy dinner recipe, which you can get ready in less than 30 minutes. Dukkah is such an easy rub to store and use when you need to make something delicious quickly. I even like it sprinkled over eggs or vegetables. Brussels sprouts were ruined when some stupid person told us to boil them; please try roasting them before you say you hate sprouts.

serves 4

2 tbsp tamari
1 tsp garlic powder
14 oz/4 cups Brussels sprouts, halved
2 tbsp sesame oil
2 garlic cloves, thinly sliced
½ red chile, seeded and finely chopped
1 small red onion, chopped
2 bok choy
½ cup slivered almonds, toasted
1 tsp coconut oil
4 x 5¼-oz organic salmon fillets
cilantro leaves, to serve

for the dukkah

3 tbsp coriander seeds
2 tbsp cumin seeds
¼ cup sesame seeds
3 cups pistachios, toasted
salt and ground black pepper, to season

1. Preheat the oven to 350°F.

2. To make the dukkah, dry fry the seeds in a small skillet over low heat for 2 minutes (until fragrant and toasted). Leave to cool, then place them in a food processor with the pistachios. Blend until the mixture is crumb-like. Season to taste and leave to one side.

3. Meanwhile, melt the coconut oil and mix with the tamari and garlic powder. Place the Brussels sprouts in a baking pan and drizzle over the oil mixture. Cook in the preheated oven for 30 minutes, until nicely roasted. Once cooked, leave to cool.

4. Heat a lidded wok over medium–high heat, add the sesame oil and, once piping hot, add the garlic, chile, and red onion. Sauté for 5 minutes, until the onion is soft. Add the bok choy and cover the wok for 2 minutes. Take off the heat. Add the Brussels sprouts and almonds. Mix well.

5. Heat the coconut oil in a large skillet. Roll the salmon in the dukkah mixture. Fry the salmon over low heat for 3 minutes each side, or until cooked to your liking (I like it slightly raw in the middle).

6. Serve with the Brussels sprout salad and a sprinkling of cilantro.

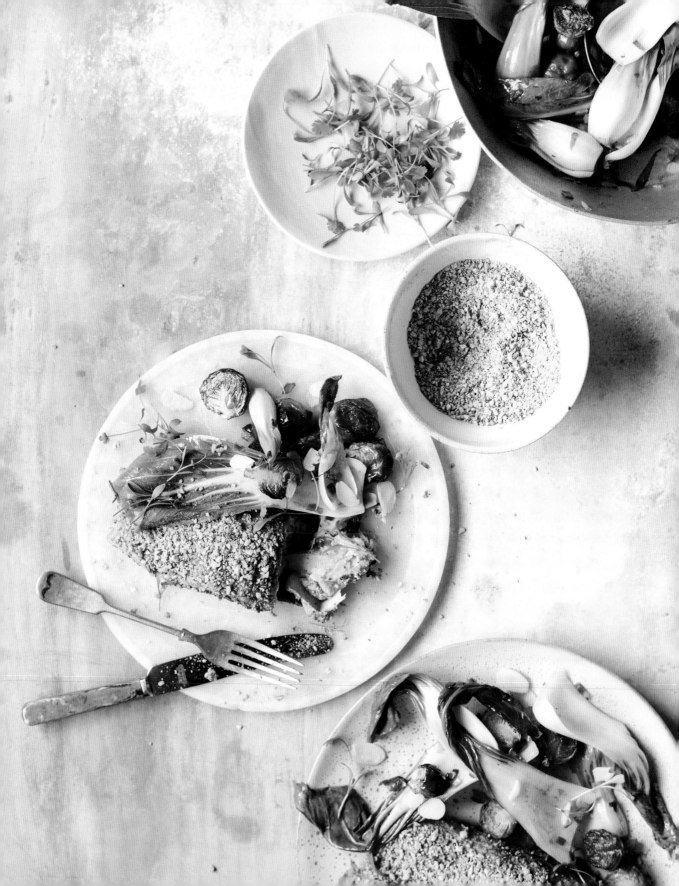

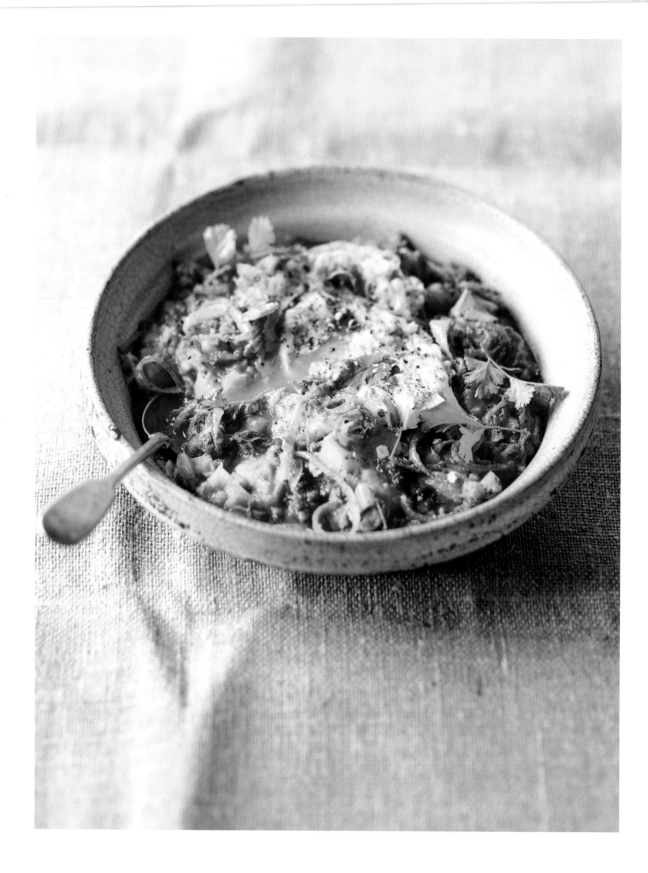

TURMERIC DAL

If a cold is brewing, or it's one of those cold wintery nights and all you want to do is put your feet up on the sofa and not spend your evening preparing dinner, this is the answer. This Turmeric Dal can sit on the stovetop simmering away for hours (getting tastier and tastier). I could eat this for breakfast, lunch, and dinner. It's great for breakfast with a fried egg on the top.

serves 4

2 cups red lentils
1 tbsp coconut oil
4 onions, sliced
8 garlic cloves, crushed
2¾ oz fresh, unpeeled ginger root, grated
half a red chile, seeded and finely chopped
1 tbsp ground coriander
1 tbsp ground cumin
1 tbsp ground turmeric
1 tsp garam masala
1 tsp ground cinnamon
2 leeks, sliced into discs
2 carrots, finely diced
2 celery stalks, finely diced
4 cups bone broth (see Miracle Bone Broth on page 159) or vegetable stock
3 large handfuls of cilantro, stalks finely chopped and leaves roughly chopped, plus extra to serve
1 tbsp tamari
large pinch of ground black pepper
1 cauliflower, cut into florets
8¾ oz/3¾ cups kale or cavolo nero, roughly chopped
juice of 1 lemon
lemon wedges, to serve

1. Wash the lentils in a colander and leave to drain.

2. Heat a large lidded saucepan and add the coconut oil. Once melted, turn the heat down to low and add the onions, garlic, ginger, and chile. Leave to sauté for 5 minutes, until the onion is soft.

3. Add the spices and mix well. Remove 4 tablespoons of the mixture to garnish the bowls before serving. Add the leeks, carrots, celery, and lentils and stir to coat with the onion mix.

4. Pour the bone broth or vegetable stock into the large saucepan and stir well.

5. Add the cilantro, tamari, and pepper and stir well. Add the cauliflower. Cover and leave to simmer for a minimum of 30 minutes, stirring the bottom of the pan occasionally to prevent sticking.

6. Once the lentils and vegetables are cooked through, add the kale or cavolo nero and mix in with the lemon juice. Add more broth or water, if needed.

7. To serve, divide the dal between 4 bowls and add a spoonful of the onion mixture and a sprinkle of cilantro leaves to each, with a wedge of fresh lemon.

STICKY CHICKEN THIGHS

This is pure comfort food. I love these chicken thighs cooked on the barbecue in the summer with a crunchy fresh salad and a big spoon of guacamole or salsa. The kids love this with the Sweet Potato Wedges and Crispy Chickpea Bake (page 191).

serves 4

5 oz tomato paste

2 tbsp honey (optional)

1 tbsp tamari

1 tbsp apple cider vinegar

1 tsp paprika

generous pinch of black pepper

1 lb 5 oz organic chicken thighs

drizzle of rapeseed/canola oil

for the salsa

4 large tomatoes

small handful of cilantro, with stalks,
    finely chopped

1 green chile, seeded and finely chopped

1 small garlic clove, finely chopped

1 small red onion, finely chopped

juice of 1 lime

salt and ground black pepper, to season

drizzle of good-quality olive oil

1. Preheat the oven to 400°F.

2. In a large bowl, mix together the tomato paste, honey (if using), tamari, apple cider vinegar, paprika, and pepper to make the marinade. Season to taste. Add the chicken thighs to the bowl and toss until each one is completely coated.

3. Put the thighs on a large baking tray. Drizzle with a little oil and bake for 20 minutes in the preheated oven, or until completely cooked through and golden brown. Turn halfway through cooking.

4. Meanwhile, make the salsa. Finely chop the tomatoes and add to a small bowl with the cilantro. Mix in the chile, garlic, onion, and lime juice. Season to taste and add a good splash of oil. Mix again and leave in the fridge until the chicken is ready.

5. Serve the thighs with sweet potato wedges, a green salad, and a big spoonful of salsa.

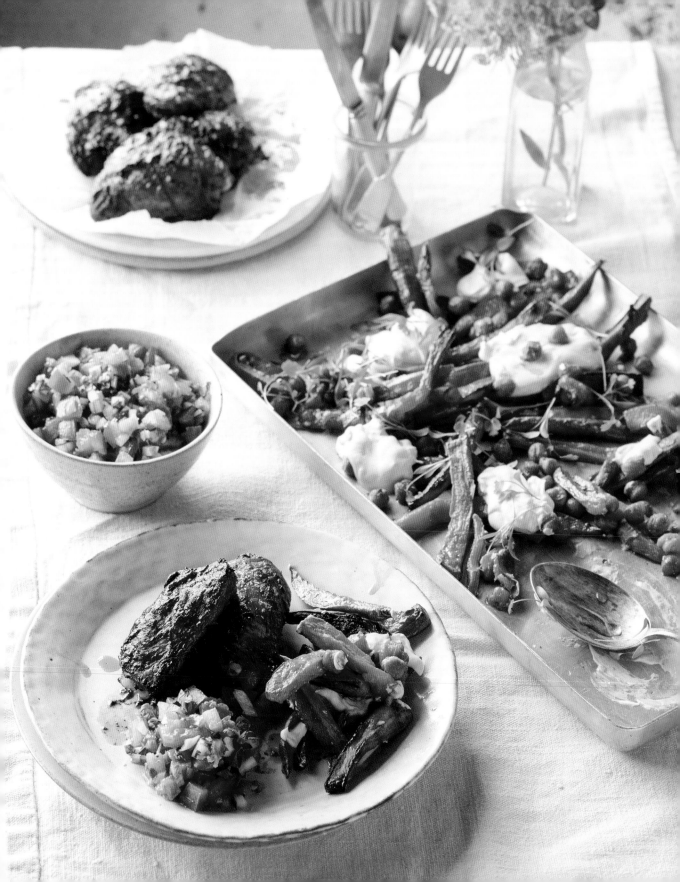

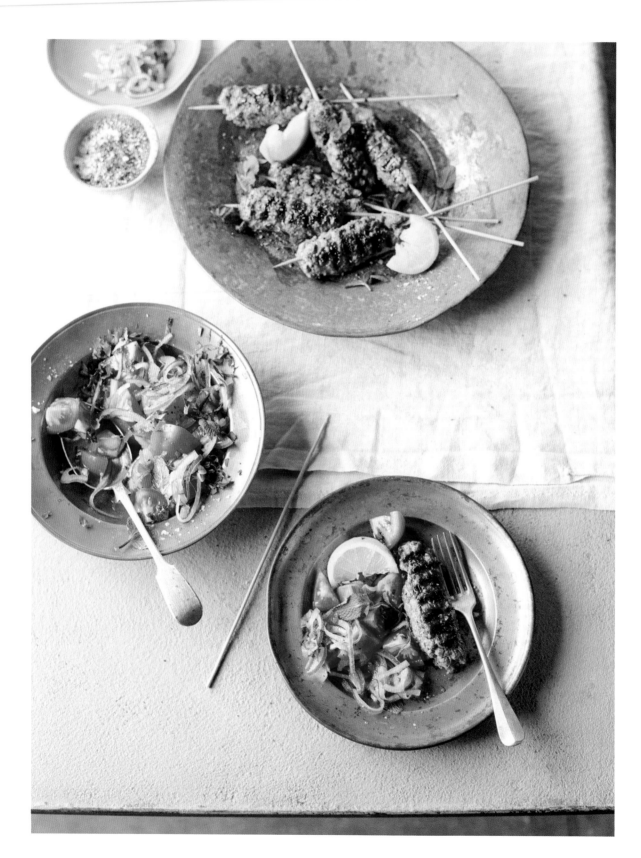

LAMB KOFTAS WITH TOMATO AND ONION SALAD

Grass-fed lamb is packed with CLA (a naturally occurring fatty acid), which helps break down stored fats in the body. It can even help reduce inflammation in the gut.

serves 4

1 lb 2 oz organic ground lamb
1 small onion, finely chopped
2 garlic cloves, crushed
1 fresh red chile, seeded and finely chopped
¾-inch piece of fresh ginger root, peeled and grated
small handful of fresh mint leaves, chopped
small handful of cilantro leaves, chopped
½ tbsp ground cumin
½ tbsp ground coriander
1 tbsp tomato paste
large pinch of Himalayan pink salt
4 tsp coconut oil, melted
lemon wedges, to serve

for the tomato and onion salad

4 tomatoes, chopped
1 red onion, chopped
4 fresh mint sprigs, chopped
2 cilantro sprigs, chopped
1 tbsp olive oil
salt and ground black pepper, to season

1. Mix together the lamb, onion, garlic, chile, ginger, herbs, spices, tomato paste, and salt in a bowl. Divide the mixture into 8 portions and roll each portion into a sausage shape. Thread each kofta onto a metal or bamboo skewer. Cover and keep in the fridge until you're ready to cook them.

2. To make the salad, mix the chopped tomatoes with the onion, mint, cilantro, and olive oil. Season to taste.

3. Heat a grill pan over medium heat. Lightly brush the koftas with the melted coconut oil. Cook them for 3–4 minutes on each side. Remove from the pan and serve with the Tomato and Onion Salad and a wedge of lemon.

Top Tip These koftas can be made in big batches and frozen. Just make sure you defrost them thoroughly before reheating.

MOROCCAN TAGINE

This is another one-pot lifesaver. Serve it with the Israeli salad from the Middle Eastern Bowl (pages 128–129) and a big spoonful of quinoa. Cook a big batch and enjoy it throughout the week.

serves 4

1 butternut squash (approximately 2¾ lbs), peeled and chopped into bite-size chunks
salt and ground black pepper
1 tbsp coconut oil, melted
1 tbsp rapeseed/canola oil
2 shallots, chopped
1 tsp ground cinnamon
3 garlic cloves, crushed
2 tbsp fresh root ginger, grated
2 red bell peppers, seeded and sliced
2 eggplants, chopped
1 x 14-oz can chickpeas (garbanzo beans), drained
1 x 14-oz can chopped tomatoes
1⅔ cups vegetable stock
4 tbsp cilantro, chopped (stalks included)
1 tbsp ras el hanout
1½ tsp ground turmeric
1 tbsp Homemade Harissa (page 185) or good-quality store-bought

1. Preheat the oven to 350°F and line a baking sheet with parchment paper.

2. Place the squash on the sheet and drizzle with coconut oil. Season with salt and pepper. Roast in the preheated oven for 25 minutes, until cooked through.

3. Once the squash is nearly cooked, heat a large, lidded saucepan over medium heat (or a tagine dish, if you are fancy) and add the rapeseed oil. Once hot, add the shallots, cinnamon, garlic, and ginger. Leave to sauté for about 5 minutes.

4. Add the bell peppers, eggplants, and roasted squash and mix well. Then add the chickpeas, canned tomatoes, vegetable stock, and the rest of the herbs and spices. Cover and leave to simmer for 20 minutes over low heat. Season to taste.

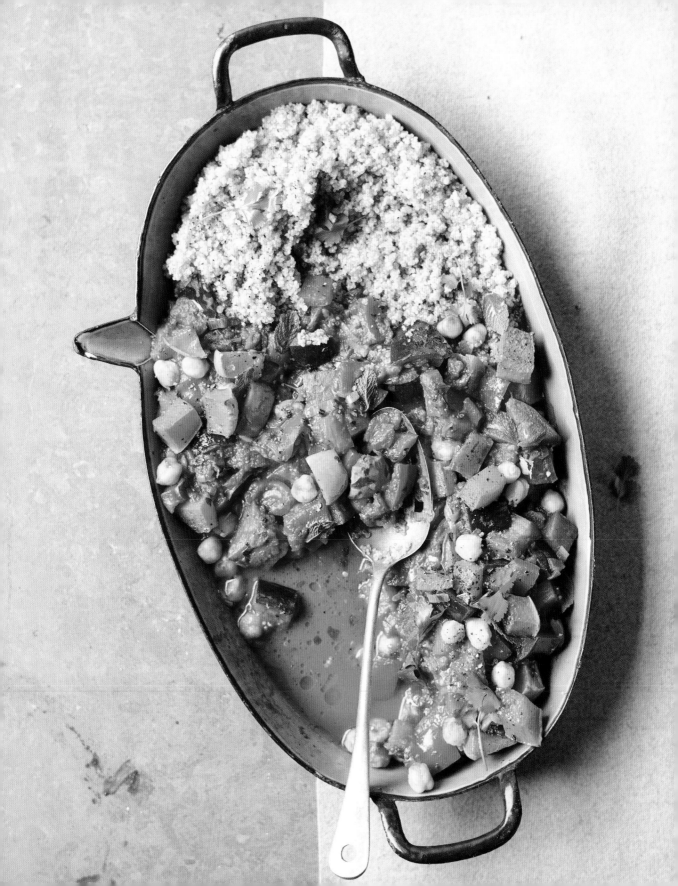

TUNA POKÉ BOWL

One of my favorite restaurants is Granger & Co., which is lucky because it is less than a 30-second walk from Bodyism, London. As often as I can, I order their life-changing Tuna Poké dish; it is such a wholesome yet fresh-tasting meal. I've tried to make a simple version for you. The marinade is one of my favorites and works well with pretty much all fish.

serves 4

¼ cup tamari
1 tsp rice vinegar
1½ tsp sesame seeds (plus extra to garnish)
¾ tsp chili flakes
4 scallions, thinly sliced
1 lb/2¼ cups sushi-grade tuna, cut into
  ¾-inch cubes
2 cups brown rice, cooked in stock
2 tomatoes, chopped
1 avocado, sliced lengthwise
small handful of cilantro, chopped
small handful of toasted coconut flakes

1. Mix the tamari, rice vinegar, sesame seeds, chili flakes, and scallions in a bowl. Add the tuna and mix well. Leave to marinate for a minimum of 2 hours in the fridge or ideally overnight.

2. Build your poké bowl. Spoon an equal amount of the rice into 4 bowls, add the tomatoes and a few slices of avocado, and the tuna. Sprinkle with cilantro and coconut flakes and serve.

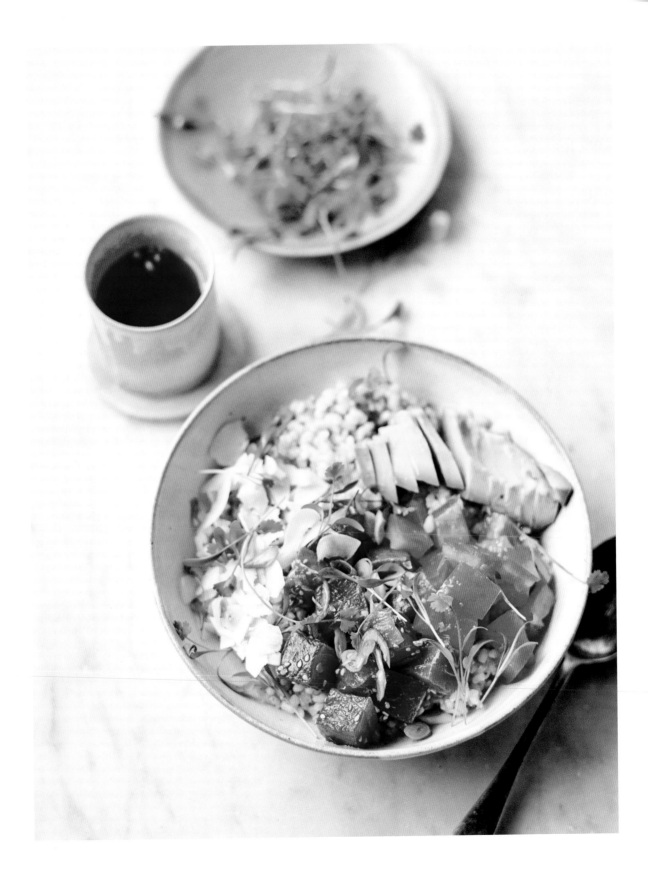

MIDDLE EASTERN MEATBALLS

The key to these meatballs is to mince all the ingredients finely with a sharp knife; this not only forms a smoother textured meatball but also makes sure they cook through evenly. Don't hold back with the herbs and spices—be guided by your own taste buds and choose whatever you like.

serves 4
1 lb ground lamb or turkey
½ tsp ground cumin
¼ tsp ground coriander
1 garlic clove, crushed
half a small red onion, finely minced
1 tsp chile, finely minced
handful of cilantro, finely chopped
handful of fresh parsley, finely chopped
1 organic, free-range egg, lightly beaten
1 tsp olive oil
1 x 14-oz can chopped tomatoes
1 tsp salt
1 tsp ground black pepper
½ tsp ground sumac
5–6 whole cabbage leaves, to serve

1. Put the meat, ground cumin, ground coriander, garlic, chile, chopped herbs, and beaten egg in a bowl. Using clean hands, mix everything together and make sure the flavorings are well distributed.

2. Again using your hands, or a big spoon, roll the mixture into medium-size balls (you should get 7–8 meatballs).

3. Heat the olive oil in a large skillet over high heat and place the meatballs in; you should hear a good sizzle when you do this.

4. Brown the meatballs for 1 minute on each side. If you feel the meat has released a lot of fat into the pan, take the meatballs out, discard the fat and put the meatballs back in.

5. Once your meatballs are brown on all sides, pour in the tomatoes and add the salt, pepper, and sumac.

6. Leave the meatballs in the tomato sauce to simmer and finish cooking for about 7 minutes. You can check if they're done by cutting into one or by pressing the meat with a finger (the meatball should feel quite firm).

7. While the meatballs are cooking, prepare the cabbage leaves. I find the easiest way is to chop the bottom root off the cabbage and pull the whole leaves off one by one.

8. Wrap each meatball, with a drizzle of sauce, in a cabbage leaf and enjoy!

SEXY STIR-FRY

We all need a dish that we can rustle up when there is nothing left in the fridge. This is so simple, delicious, healthy, and quick. Use up whatever veggies you have lying around—it doesn't have to be the combination listed below. Add shrimp or thinly sliced chicken to increase the protein. The eggs make this meal more substantial; if you don't want them scrambled, serve them fried, on top of the noodles, with a few cilantro leaves and a grind of fresh pepper.

serves 4

7 oz flat, wide rice noodles

2 tbsp tamari or soy sauce

½ tbsp honey

1½ tbsp freshly squeezed lime juice, plus an extra squeeze, to serve

1 tbsp coconut, vegetable, or olive oil, plus extra for scrambling the eggs

1 carrot, peeled and finely sliced into discs

1 red or yellow bell pepper, finely sliced lengthwise

1 small zucchini, peeled and finely sliced into discs

1 tsp finely minced fresh chile, or dried chili flakes

2 garlic cloves, finely minced

1 tsp finely minced fresh ginger root

2 organic, free-range eggs, whisked

1 tbsp sesame seeds

handful of cilantro, roughly chopped

1. First, soak the noodles in a bowl of hot water; they can soften while you get the rest of the ingredients ready. They should soften up in under 10 minutes.

2. Mix the tamari or soy sauce, honey, and lime juice in a bowl.

3. Put a large skillet over high heat and pour in the oil. Let it heat up and then throw in the carrots to cook for a minute, followed by the bell peppers. Let them sauté and get some color for about 2 minutes on the high heat and then add in the zucchini, chile (if using fresh), garlic, and ginger. Stir everything around and cook for 2 minutes.

4. Now pour over the tamari, honey, and lime juice sauce and mix everything together well.

5. Transfer everything from the pan to a plate or bowl.

6. Drain the noodles.

7. Add a small splash of oil to the pan and pour in the whisked eggs with a pinch of salt and pepper (remember the tamari/soy is salty).

8. Whisk the eggs and, when they start to scramble, add the noodles and stir them into the egg mixture.

9. Add the rest of your ingredients back in, mix everything together, adding your dried chili flakes now, if using.

10. Add a final squeeze of lime, top with the sesame seeds and cilantro, and serve.

SLOW-COOKED IRISH STEW

This dish is not only comforting and hearty, it is also really healthy and a great cold-buster. Stews are about building layers of flavor, so take the time to do each step properly and enjoy the process. Get organized and prep your vegetables and garlic beforehand—then it's super simple.

serves 4

1 tbsp olive oil
1½ lbs lamb neck, cubed
1 white onion, finely minced
2 large garlic cloves, finely minced
3 carrots, peeled and chopped
1 large parsnip, peeled and chopped
large handful of cavolo nero or kale,
    chopped (stalks discarded)
2 bay leaves
a few sprigs of thyme
1 rosemary stalk
½ tsp salt
½ tsp ground black pepper
5 baby potatoes, chopped (optional)

1. Preheat the oven to 350°F.

2. First comes browning the meat, which gives color and seals in flavor. In a large, lidded casserole dish or ovenproof stockpot, heat half of the olive oil over high heat. Add in the meat. If there isn't enough room in your pot for each meat piece to have contact with the bottom of the pan to brown, do it in batches. Do the first side for 2 minutes and then turn. You should hear a good sizzle when the meat hits the pan.

3. Once browned, take all the meat out of the pot and set aside. Turn down the heat to medium and add in the rest of the olive oil.

4. Add in the onion and stir. Try to scrape up any brown bits at the bottom of the pan from the meat, because these are full of flavor. Once the onion is translucent, after about 2 minutes, add in the garlic and cook for another minute.

5. Add in the carrots, parsnip, kale, bay leaves, and herbs and add half the salt and pepper. Stir everything together.

6. Put all the meat back in the pot and pour in enough boiling water to cover the meat.

7. Add the remaining salt and pepper and stir everything together. If using the potatoes, let them just rest on top of the meat and water. Put a lid on the pot and put it into the preheated oven for at least 2½ hours, or 3 if you have the time.

8. Serve up into bowls and enjoy.

MIRACLE BONE BROTH

This incredible bone broth is packed with antioxidants and collagen, making it a truly healthy elixir. You can use leftover bones from a Sunday roast or ask the butcher — often they'll give them to you for free! Make sure you're using collagen-rich bones, like marrow, knuckles, and feet, from organic lamb or chicken.

This recipe has a few steps, but nothing complicated and the result is so worth it. It also makes quite a bit of broth, so you can freeze some and keep the rest in your fridge for up to 4 days. Feel free to drink a cup on its own or add it to curries and pasta sauces and use as a stock base for soups for a nutritional boost.

Start your broth in the morning—you'll want to leave it simmering over low heat for up to 12 hours to get maximum nourishment from the bones. At room temperature, it has a jelly-like consistency. If it looks strange—you've made it correctly.

serves 4, with leftovers

2¼ lbs organic lamb or chicken bones
   (marrow, knuckles, feet, or other
   collagen-rich bones)
3 onions, skin on, chopped in half
3 carrots, chopped in half
5 garlic cloves, smashed
4 bay leaves
½ tbsp peppercorns
½ tsp salt
½ tbsp apple cider vinegar

1. Preheat the oven to 400°F.

2. Put the bones in a large stockpot and fill with cold water; bring to a boil over high heat and let it boil for about 20 minutes. This initial step removes all the impurities from the bones and is called blanching.

3. Discard the water, put the bones in a roasting pan and place in the oven to caramelize for about an hour. This enhances the depth of flavor in the broth and starts breaking down the collagen in the bones.

4. Return the bones to your pot, together with the onions, carrots, garlic, bay leaves, peppercorns, salt, and cider vinegar, and refill with (preferably filtered) water. These few additional ingredients add an aromatic quality to your broth and really deepen the flavor.

5. Bring up to a boil, then turn down and leave to simmer for as long as you can—preferably up to 12 hours to really get the maximum nutrition out of the bones and develop a flavorsome broth.

6. To finish, pour the broth through a fine-mesh strainer into a wide and shallow container, which will help the broth cool down quicker. All the fat will rise to the top once the broth cools; skim the fat off and either discard it or use it for other recipes.

7. Once cool, refrigerate or freeze.

POACHED COCONUT CHICKEN AND CAULI-RICE

This is a quick, easy, and fuss-free dinner. If using a box grater for the cauliflower, do it on top of the baking sheet in which you plan to roast it to save on mess.

serves 2

2 organic chicken breasts (approximately
    5¼ oz each)
1 cauliflower
¼ tsp salt
¼ tsp ground black pepper
½ tbsp coconut oil, melted
1 lemongrass stalk
1 x 14-fl oz can coconut milk
half a small red chile
¾-inch piece of fresh ginger root
½ tbsp fish sauce
1 red or yellow bell pepper, julienned
handful of cilantro, chopped
juice of 1 lime

1. Preheat the oven to 375°F.

2. Let the chicken come to room temperature while you prepare the other ingredients.

3. Either grate the whole head of cauliflower with a box grater or place it in a food processor and pulse to small rice-size pieces. Sprinkle with half the salt and pepper and pour over the coconut oil.

4. Mix with your hands and spread thinly on a baking sheet. Put into the preheated oven and leave to roast for 20 minutes. After about 10 minutes, give it a toss.

5. Crush the lemongrass stalk with the back of a spoon a few times to bruise it and release its aroma. Pour the coconut milk into a medium–hot pan and add the lemongrass, chile, ginger, and fish sauce. Let it simmer for approximately 3 minutes.

6. Sprinkle both chicken breasts with the remaining salt and pepper. Add the chicken and bell pepper to the pan of simmering sauce. Turn both breasts after 5 minutes and do the same again 5 minutes later. The chicken should be cooked in just under 15 minutes.

7. Take the chicken out and cover in foil. Turn up the heat in the pan and boil the sauce to reduce and thicken it for about 3 minutes. Shred the chicken with a fork and add it back into the sauce.

8. Divide the cauli-rice between two plates and spoon the chicken on top. Sprinkle over the chopped cilantro and add a final squeeze of lime. Eat up!

KERALAN FISH CURRY

The subtle heat in this dish comes from the green chile and ginger, while the spices bring a warm depth to the dish that is hard to describe but it is absolutely delicious.

serves 4, with leftovers

for the masala

1 tbsp coriander seeds

1 tsp cumin seeds

2 star anise

1 tsp ground turmeric

3 garlic cloves, finely minced

half a small green chile, seeded and chopped

1 tsp salt

1-inch piece of fresh ginger root, peeled and grated or finely minced

for the dish

1½ tbsp vegetable, coconut, or olive oil

1 red onion, finely chopped

1 large tomato, chopped into small chunks

½ tsp white vinegar

½ cup hot water

1 x 14-fl oz can coconut milk

14 oz firm white fish, like cod or pollock, cut into even-size chunks

7 oz shrimp

¼ tsp freshly ground black pepper

pinch of salt

juice of half a lime

large handful of cilantro, roughly chopped

1. Make the masala first. Toast the spices in a hot, dry pan to release their flavors. Grind the spices into a powder in a food processor or coffee grinder and mix in the garlic, chile, salt, and ginger.

2. Heat 1 tablespoon of the oil in a medium–hot skillet and sauté the onion for about 2 minutes, until softened. Add in the masala paste and let it cook for a few minutes, until you can really smell the spices, and the garlic, ginger, and chile are cooked.

3. Add in the chopped tomatoes and the vinegar and let everything cook in the pan for a minute.

4. Add the hot water and let the whole mix simmer for about 5 minutes.

5. If you're making brown rice or quinoa to accompany this dish, now is the time to get it going in another pan. Follow the package instructions and, if cooking quinoa, be sure to put a lid on the pan to cook the grain properly and, once done, cover with a dish towel to allow it to continue steaming. This makes for light, airy quinoa.

6. After 5 minutes of the masala mix simmering, add in the can of coconut milk and stir everything together.

7. Add in the fish, shrimp, pepper, and salt. Simmer for about 7 minutes, until the fish is cooked.

8. Squeeze the lime juice into the pan and toss in the cilantro. Taste the sauce to see if it needs more lime, salt, or pepper. Serve up with brown rice, quinoa, or your grains of choice!

PERFECT ROAST CHICKEN

Everyone needs a roast chicken recipe up their sleeve. It is truly one of the most delicious, nourishing, and comforting meals ever and will see you through so many dinners and special occasions. It's worth investing in a beautiful, organic, free-range bird; yes, it's more expensive, but one chicken can stretch into two or three meals. Not only will you have leftovers, but you can turn the carcass into delicious and healthy stock to make tasty soups (page 167), pasta sauces ... the list goes on.

serves 4

1 tsp olive oil
1 x 4-lb 3 oz chicken
½ tsp ground Himalayan pink salt
½ tsp freshly ground black pepper
half a lemon
half an onion
a few garlic cloves, smashed
a few sprigs of thyme or rosemary (use
    whichever herbs you have)

1. Preheat the oven to 400°F and allow at least 15 minutes for it to heat up properly.

2. Pour the olive oil over the chicken and sprinkle with the salt and pepper, including the cavity. Using your hands, rub the seasoning into the chicken skin.

3. Put the lemon, onion, garlic, and herbs into the chicken cavity. This will give the chicken a lovely flavor as it cooks.

4. Put the chicken into a roasting pan and cook in the preheated oven for 1 hour.

5. Take the chicken out, baste with the liquid that's in the bottom of the pan and cover with foil.

6. Let it rest for at least 10 minutes; this allows all the juices to go back into the chicken, making the bird tender and delicious.

7. Use this time, while the chicken rests, to crisp up any vegetables you have roasting or to prepare a salad. Slice, serve, and enjoy.

Top Tip If you're making stock, just simmer the chicken carcass in a large pot of water with any vegetable scraps and herbs you have in the fridge and plenty of salt and pepper for 2 hours—it's so simple and satisfying.

CHICKEN SCHNITZEL WITH ROOT VEGETABLE MASH

Who said healthy food couldn't include comfort food? This is such a warming, hearty, and healthy dinner, and it's one of Chrissy's and my favorites. Enjoy it with some delicious wholegrain mustard and a side of sautéed greens.

serves 2

for the mash
6⅔ oz/1⅓ cups butternut squash, chopped
1 tbsp coconut oil, melted
half a cauliflower, chopped (you can use the stalk)
½ cup almond milk
3 garlic cloves, crushed
1 tbsp wholegrain mustard
Himalayan pink salt and ground black pepper, to season

for the schnitzel
2 tbsp arrowroot flour
2 tbsp chickpea/gram flour
1 tsp garlic powder
1 organic, free-range egg, beaten
2 small organic chicken breasts (approximately 5¼ oz each)
1 tbsp coconut oil

1. Preheat the oven to 350°F and line a baking sheet with parchment paper.

2. Place the butternut squash on the baking sheet and drizzle with oil. Roast in the oven for 30 minutes.

3. Meanwhile, steam the cauliflower for 5 minutes or until it is very tender.

4. In a food processor, blend the roasted squash, almond milk, crushed garlic cloves, and cauliflower. Stir in the wholegrain mustard and season well.

5. For the schnitzel, mix the flours together with a pinch of salt and pepper and the garlic powder. Divide the flour mixture into two bowls. Pour the egg into a third.

6. Cover a work surface with a piece of plastic wrap. Place the chicken breasts on top and cover with another piece of plastic wrap. Using a rolling pin, bash each chicken breast until they are approximately ⅛-inch thick.

7. Dip the chicken into the flour to coat and then dip it into the egg mix and then into the last bowl of flour to coat, ensuring an even layer on each side.

8. Put the mash into a saucepan and cook over low heat, until warm and ready to serve.

9. Heat the coconut oil in a large skillet over medium heat and leave to get piping hot. Fry the chicken for 3 minutes, until crisp and crunchy on the underside. Carefully turn it and cook for another 2–3 minutes, until cooked through. Serve the schnitzel with the mash and some sautéed greens.

THE PERFECT BURGER

There are three secrets to the perfect burger. The first is to make sure the garlic and onion are really finely chopped so they mix well with the meat and cook through properly. The second is to make sure your meat mixture isn't too wet, or else the burgers won't hold together. When adding the egg, pour in half of it first and mix with your hands; if the mixture feels like it will come together and form nice patties, then leave the other half of the whisked egg out. The third is to make sure you have properly seasoned the raw meat for fantastic flavor. Now, go on, steal my secrets and make a damn tasty burger!

serves 4

1 garlic clove, finely chopped
handful of finely chopped red onion
handful of fresh parsley, finely chopped
1 lb 2 oz ground lamb
½ tsp salt
½ tsp ground black pepper
½ tbsp Dijon or wholegrain mustard
1 organic, free-range egg, beaten
½ tbsp olive oil

1. Put the garlic, onion, and parsley into a bowl with the meat. Season the meat with the salt and black pepper.

2. Add the mustard and pour in half the beaten egg. Mix it all together with your hands and judge whether the mix could do with more egg or if it will form firm burger patties without it.

3. Form the mixture into 4 large burger patties or 6 smaller ones, bearing in mind that the smaller ones will take less time to cook.

4. Heat a large skillet over high heat and, once hot, add the oil. Let it get hot (this will take 1–2 minutes).

5. Add the burgers to the pan; you should hear a sizzle when you do this—if not, the pan isn't hot enough and the burgers will taste bland. Sear the burgers for about 4 minutes on each side. Test the meat with your finger; it should feel firm and a little springy to the touch for medium doneness. You could finish them in a hot oven for another few minutes, if you like your meat well done, but I think this dries the burgers out and ruins the texture.

6. Take off the heat and leave to rest for 1–2 minutes before serving; this allows all the juices to run back into the middle of the burger, keeping it moist and juicy—enjoy!

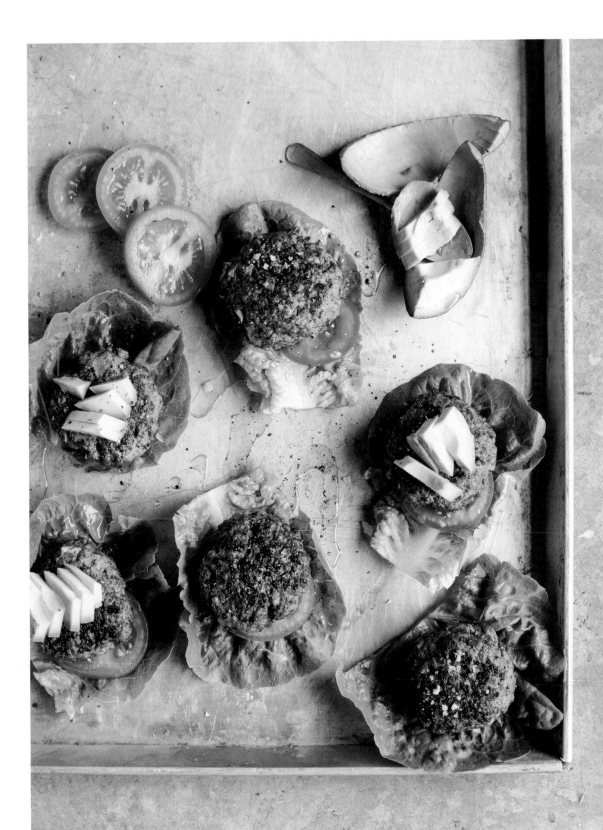

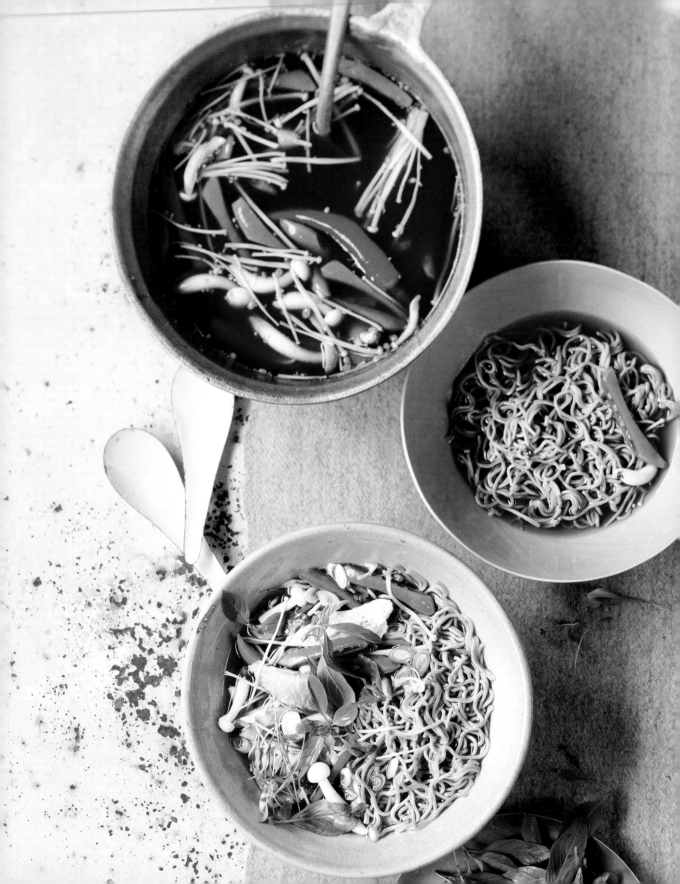

LEFTOVER ROAST CHICKEN PHO

I always make this after we've had a roast, because it's a delicious way of using up leftovers. The tangy flavors of the tamari and brown-rice miso are so tasty. If you want an extra protein boost, enjoy it with a soft-boiled egg!

serves 4

1 whole organic corn-fed, free-range chicken carcass (it's best to make this soup after you make Perfect Roast Chicken, on page 162)

2 cups organic chicken stock

1 whole red chile

thumb of fresh ginger root, grated

1 lemongrass stalk, crushed

1 tbsp tamari

1 tbsp organic apple cider vinegar

1 tbsp brown-rice miso paste

1 tbsp fish sauce

8 oz buckwheat soba noodles

5¼ oz/1½ cups sugar snap peas

3 cups sliced mushrooms

4 tbsp scallions, thinly sliced

4 tbsp cilantro, roughly chopped, to garnish

1. In a large stockpot, combine the chicken carcass with the chicken stock, bring to a boil and simmer over low heat for at least an hour. Remove from the heat; the remaining chicken meat should have fallen off the bone. Strain through a strainer and discard the bones, returning the meat to the reserved liquid. Put back over low heat and add the chile, ginger, lemongrass, tamari, vinegar, brown-rice miso, and fish sauce. Simmer while you prepare the soba noodles.

2. Cook the soba noodles according to the package instructions, keeping them on the al dente side. When they are cooked, rinse them immediately with cold water; this will prevent them from getting soggy.

3. Add the sugar snap peas and mushrooms to the stockpot and simmer for 15 minutes.

4. To serve, distribute the soba noodles into 4 soup bowls and top with ladles of the stock. Garnish with scallions and cilantro.

SHRIMP SUMMER ROLLS WITH TAMARI DIPPING SAUCE

These rolls are such a delicious appetizer for a dinner party. If you want to get really fancy, buy some edible flowers to add into the roll. As always, use this recipe as a guide and feel free to experiment. Swap the shrimp for chicken or more vegetables; choose whatever makes you happy!

makes 10

1 tsp butter or olive oil

1 garlic clove, crushed

10 fresh jumbo shrimp

10 rice paper rolls

half a cucumber, cut lengthwise and finely sliced lengthwise

1 whole red bell pepper, finely sliced lengthwise

3 scallions, finely sliced lengthwise

5 radishes, finely sliced

handful of cilantro, chopped

juice of 2 limes

for the dipping sauce

5 tbsp tamari

3 tbsp tahini

juice of 1 lemon

salt and ground black pepper, to taste

1. Heat the butter or oil over medium heat in a small skillet. Add the garlic and the shrimp and fry until golden on both sides; this takes 5–10 minutes. Remove from the heat and set aside. Slice each shrimp in half, so you have 20 shrimp halves to put in the rolls.

2. Fill a large bowl with boiling hot water and dip the first rice paper roll into it, until it is translucent.

3. Put the roll on a plate and put 2 shrimp halves face down on top, with 3 pieces each of cucumber, bell pepper, scallion, and radish.

4. Garnish with 1 teaspoon of the chopped cilantro and drizzle ¼ teaspoon of lime juice over the top.

5. Fold the outer edges in and roll into a small parcel.

6. Repeat for all the rolls.

7. To make the dipping sauce, combine all the ingredients in a small pitcher and mix until well combined. Pour into a bowl to dip the rolls in.

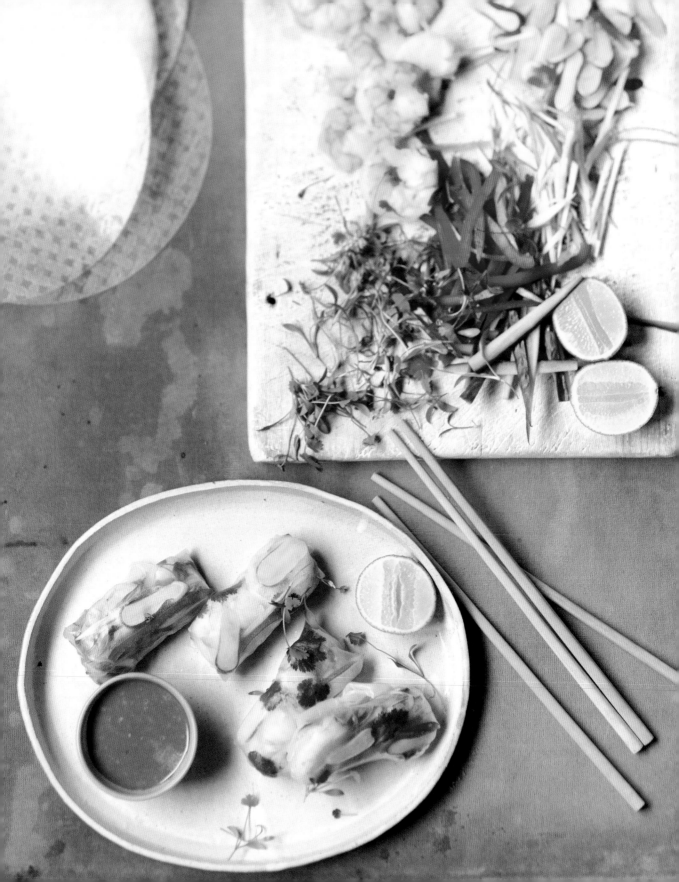

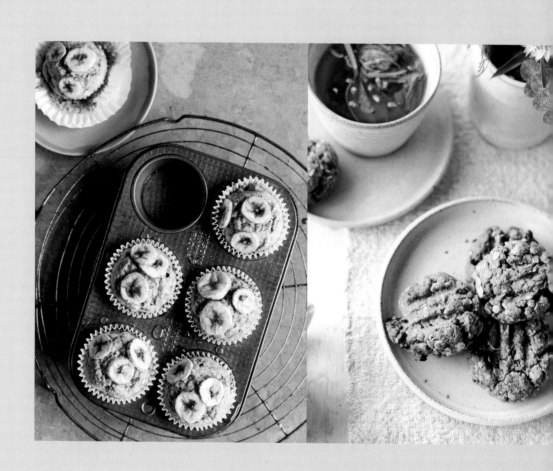

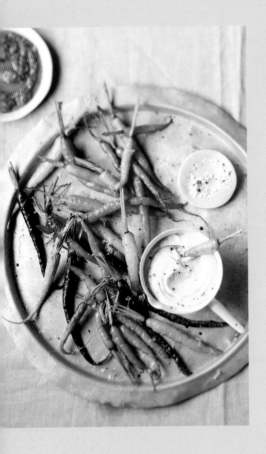

SNACKS AND SIDES

Pistachio and Raspberry Medicine Balls

Trail Mix

Pecan Salted Chocolate Bark

Not-ella

Bodyism Cookies

Almond Butter Jam Muffins

Bodyism Banana Muffins

Hummus with Harissa and Roasted Carrot Dippers

Guacamole

Rosemary Parsnip Fries

Muhammara (Roasted Red Pepper Dip)

Homemade Harissa

Whole Roasted Cauliflower

Hearty Roasted Carrots and Avocado

Sumac Fattoush

Sweet Potato Wedges and Crispy Chickpea Bake

PISTACHIO AND RASPBERRY MEDICINE BALLS

I really don't like when energy balls are marketed as "healthy" but are filled with loads of fake sugars. That's why I try to experiment with other ways of sweetening our energy balls—things like pumpkin or berries, or good fats such as coconut butter or nut butter. This ingredient list makes me smile because it's full of nourishing, wonderful ingredients.

makes 20

1 cup almonds
¾ oz coconut oil, melted
¾ cup frozen raspberries
¾ oz chia seeds
2 tbsp almond butter
1⅓ cups dried shredded coconut (plus extra, for sprinkling)
⅓ cup hemp seeds
⅓ cup buckwheat groats
1 scoop Bodyism Protein Excellence
3½ oz raw chocolate (optional, for dipping)

1. Put the almonds in a food processor and blend into a breadcrumb texture. Add the rest of the ingredients and blend until everything is well combined.

2. Use your hands to roll the mixture into walnut-size balls.

3. Roll the balls in the coconut, then place in an airtight container and stick them in the freezer for a minimum of 30 minutes. Enjoy them straight out of the freezer.

4. If you want to make these extra indulgent, melt some raw chocolate and dip the balls in the chocolate before placing them in the freezer.

TRAIL MIX

This is my go-to when I'm traveling. I don't know what it is about flying, but I'm always hungry on the plane. This very easy Trail Mix is a great way to keep satisfied and happy during your travels. Also, it's a great topping for the Açai Bowl (page 96), Protein Pancakes (page 105) or Three-Grain Oatmeal (page 100).

makes 1 lb 2 oz

2 tbsp coconut oil
2½ tsp vanilla powder
1½ cups almonds
½ cup pumpkin seeds
⅔ cup coconut flakes
¾ cup slivered almonds
⅓ cup mulberries
½ cup goji berries or bittersweet
   chocolate chips

1. Preheat the oven to 350°F and line a baking sheet with parchment paper.

2. Melt the coconut oil and stir in the vanilla powder.

3. Place the almonds, pumpkin seeds, coconut flakes, and slivered almonds in a bowl and mix in the melted coconut oil and vanilla. Stir until everything is covered.

4. Pour the mix onto the lined baking sheet, place in the preheated oven, and bake for about 20 minutes, until the almonds darken and the coconut flakes have turned golden brown.

5. Once cooked, take the mix out of the oven, leave to cool, and then stir in the mulberries and goji berries or bittersweet chocolate chips.

6. Place in an airtight container and enjoy whenever you need a healthy snack on the go.

PECAN SALTED CHOCOLATE BARK

I always thought making my own chocolate wouldn't be worth the fuss, but this recipe is so simple and makes a much tastier treat than any store-bought one. It's also perfect for wrapping up and giving as a healthy gift. I like to play around with flavor combinations, but the Pecan Salted Chocolate Bark is always my favorite.

serves 4

1 cup pecans
½ tbsp coconut oil
⅔ cup maple syrup
1 tbsp ground cinnamon
¾ cup cacao butter
¾ cup raw cacao powder
2 pinches of sea salt flakes

1. Preheat the oven to 300°F and line 2 baking pans with parchment paper. Pour the pecans into the first pan.

2. Meanwhile, melt the coconut oil in a saucepan over low heat with ¼ cup of the maple syrup and the cinnamon, stirring until well combined.

3. Pour the mixture over the pecans and mix until all the pecans are covered. Pop them into the preheated oven for 10 minutes, until they are golden.

4. Melt the cacao butter in a bowl set over boiling water; make sure the bowl isn't touching the water, and stir until completely melted. Take off the heat and rest.

5. Mix the cacao powder into the melted cacao butter and keep stirring for 3–4 minutes, until the mixture thickens up—this is the most important part of the recipe, so keep at it until it feels thick and has the consistency of melted chocolate.

6. Pour the chocolate mixture into the second baking pan, so it's about ½-inch thick. Sprinkle the pecans into the chocolate, pressing them down to make sure they are completely set into it. Sprinkle sea salt on top and place in the freezer for 2 hours.

7. Take the chocolate out and break it up into sections, however big or small you like. I keep my chocolate in the freezer in an airtight container, because it retains all the flavor and has a semifreddo-type consistency. However, keeping it in the fridge is perfectly fine, too.

NOT-ELLA

You all know about my Nutella addiction. This is my healthier version, which Chrissy has to hide when it's in the house—otherwise my addiction might reappear and you'll find me in a bath of healthy nut butter ...

makes 1 jar

1⅔ cups raw hazelnuts
2 tbsp water
2 tbsp maple syrup (optional)
1 tbsp cacao powder
1 tsp vanilla extract
½ tsp sea salt
2 tbsp cacao nibs

1. Preheat the oven to 350°F.

2. Place the hazelnuts on a baking sheet and let roast for 5–7 minutes, until toasted. Remove and let cool.

3. Place the hazelnuts in a food processor and blend on medium speed for about 10 minutes, until a paste forms. Stop every few minutes to scrape the nuts from the blade.

4. Add the remaining ingredients (apart from the cacao nibs) and pulse for a few more minutes.

5. Sprinkle the cacao nibs on top so that when you transfer the mixture to a jar they are distributed throughout. Enjoy!

BODYISM COOKIES

These cookies have their own fan club. When we've run out of them at our café in West London, protests have started. Seriously, these cookies are pretty damn good. That's why I've given you a recipe that makes 18, because they disappear before your very eyes. If you want to be smart, freeze half of the dough and, when you fancy another batch, just defrost and roll it out. Drum roll, please..

makes 18–20

1⅓ cups oat flour (or gluten-free oats blended to a fine powder in a food processor)
½ cup coconut flour
2¼ cups gluten-free oats
½ tsp baking soda
1 cup plus 2 tbsp coconut palm sugar
1 tsp Himalayan pink salt
2 tsp vanilla extract
¾ cup coconut oil, melted
3 organic, free-range eggs, beaten
3½ oz/⅔ cup sugar-free bittersweet chocolate, cut into small squares

1. Preheat the oven to 400°F and line 2 baking sheets with parchment paper.

2. In a large mixing bowl, mix the flours, oats, baking soda, sugar, and salt together.

3. In another bowl, mix the vanilla extract and coconut oil together.

4. Slowly mix the liquid mixture into the dry mixture. Then slowly stir in the beaten eggs.

5. Finally, add the chocolate, and, using your hands, mix it in.

6. Roll 1 dessertspoon of the cookie dough into a small ball and place on a baking sheet. Repeat this step until you've used up all the mixture, making sure you leave quite a bit of space between each ball.

7. Using the back of a fork, flatten each ball.

8. Bake in the oven for 12–15 minutes, until golden brown. Then let cool (remember they cook more as they cool down).

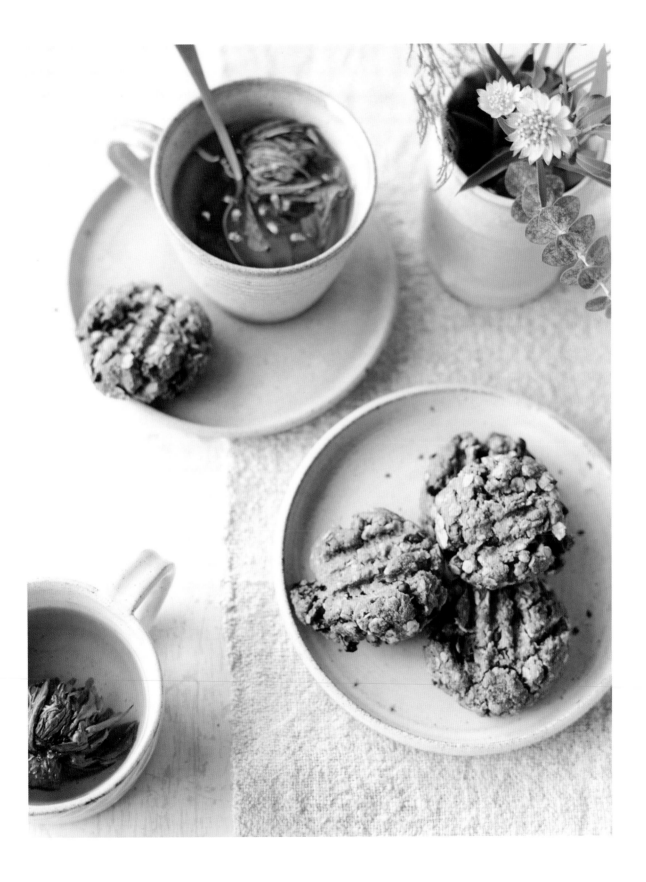

ALMOND BUTTER JAM MUFFINS

Muffins can be the most delicious, indulgent snack in the world—or the biggest disappointment. These muffins are really gooey and the almond butter and jam give them the perfect balance of salty and sweet.

makes 12

1 cup pecans
2 organic, free-range eggs, beaten
⅓ cup maple syrup
¼ cup coconut palm sugar
¼ cup coconut oil, melted
¾ cup applesauce
½ cup almond butter
pinch of sea salt
1½ tsp baking powder
½ tsp baking soda
1 tsp apple cider vinegar
¼ cup almond milk
½ cup quinoa flour
½ cup buckwheat flour
½ cup ground almonds
¾ cup gluten-free oats
6 tsp sugar-free strawberry jam

1. Preheat the oven to 350°F and line a standard muffin pan with 12 muffin liners.

2. Pour the eggs into a mixing bowl, add the maple syrup, coconut sugar, and oil, and whisk well.

3. Add the applesauce, almond butter, salt, baking powder, baking soda, and apple cider vinegar and whisk to combine.

4. Add the almond milk and whisk again to combine.

5. Lastly, add the flours, ground almonds, and oats and whisk or stir until just combined.

6. Spoon the mixture into the muffin liners until they are half full. Then add half a teaspoon of the strawberry jam to each. Add a tablespoon more mixture on top of the jam, to cover it.

7. Place in the preheated oven and cook for 25 minutes, until a toothpick inserted into the center of one of the muffins comes out clean.

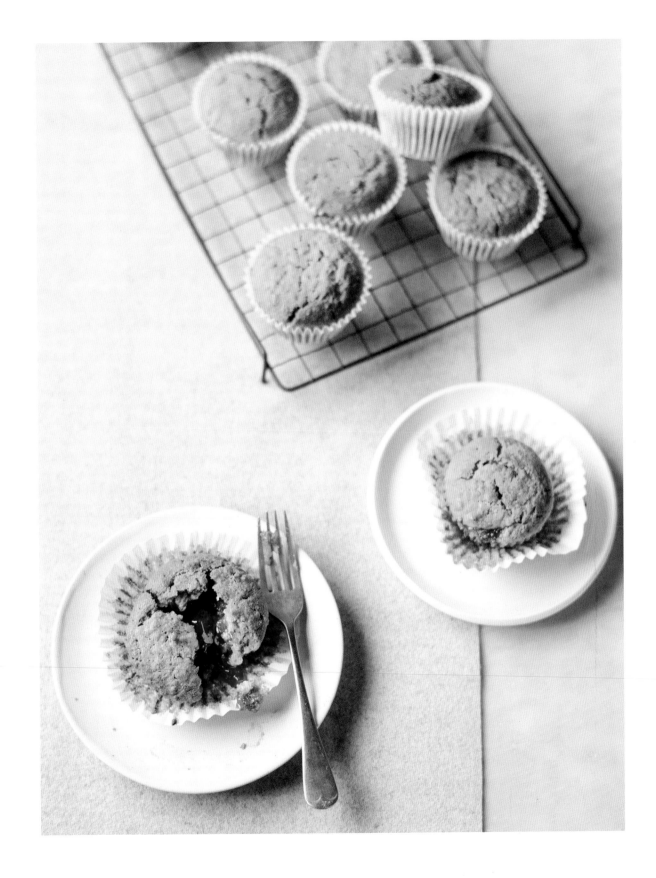

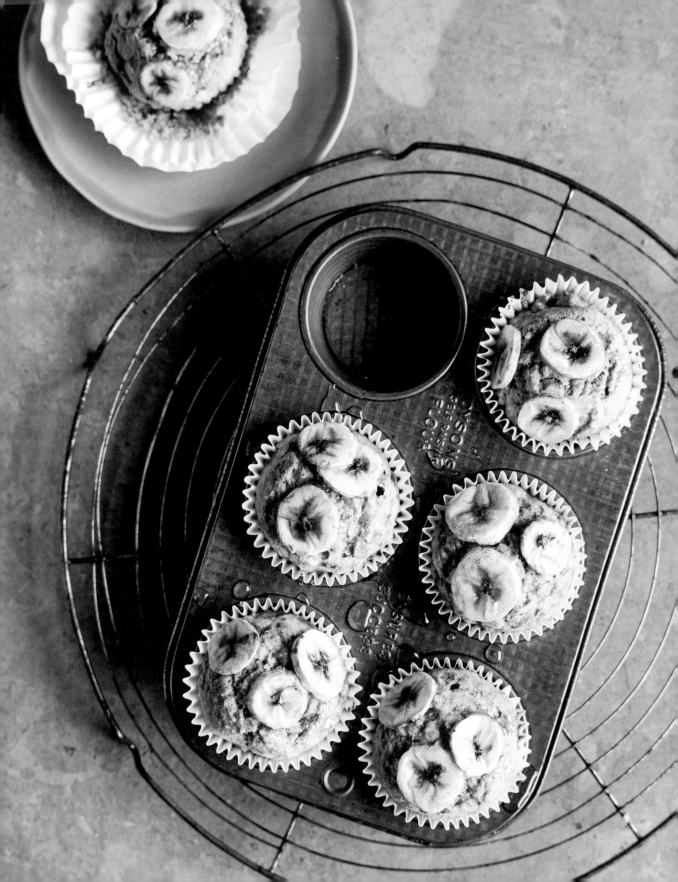

BODYISM BANANA MUFFINS

The flour mix that we use in this recipe is our go-to for any cake. The different flours make the perfect gluten-free replacement for starchy all-purpose flour. Just mix it up and keep the leftovers to make any other gluten-free cake that takes your fancy.

makes 12

1 cup plus 2 tbsp gluten-free flour mix (see below)
6 tbsp almond flour
1 tsp baking powder
¾ tsp Himalayan pink salt
½ tsp ground cinnamon
3 tbsp flaxseeds
3 tbsp roughly chopped walnuts, toasted
6 tbsp coconut oil, melted
6 tbsp maple syrup
6 tbsp coconut milk
2 tbsp almond butter
2 tsp vanilla extract
6 ripe bananas (4 mashed, 2 sliced)

for the gluten-free flour mix

2¾ cups brown rice flour
1¾ cups oat flour (or gluten-free oats blended to a fine powder in a food processor)
1¾ cups coconut flour
½ cup tapioca flour

1. Preheat the oven to 350°F and line a 12-cup muffin pan with 12 paper liners or 2 x 6-cup muffin pans with 6 paper liners each.

2. In a large bowl, mix together the flour mix, almond flour, baking powder, salt, cinnamon, and flaxseeds to remove any lumps. Stir in the walnuts.

3. In a small bowl, combine the oil, 5 tablespoons of the maple syrup, the coconut milk, almond butter, and vanilla. Whisk to combine. Fold in the mashed bananas.

4. Pour the wet mixture into the dry mixture and whisk together by hand, until just combined.

5. Lightly toss the sliced bananas with the remaining maple syrup.

6 Fill the muffin cups almost all the way up and top with 3 banana slices per muffin.

7. Bake for 35–40 minutes in the preheated oven, until the muffins have browned and spring back slightly to the touch.

Top Tip Whenever you eat fruit, try to eat it with a good fat, because it slows down the absorption of the sugar so that you don't have a sugar spike and become moody for the rest of the afternoon.

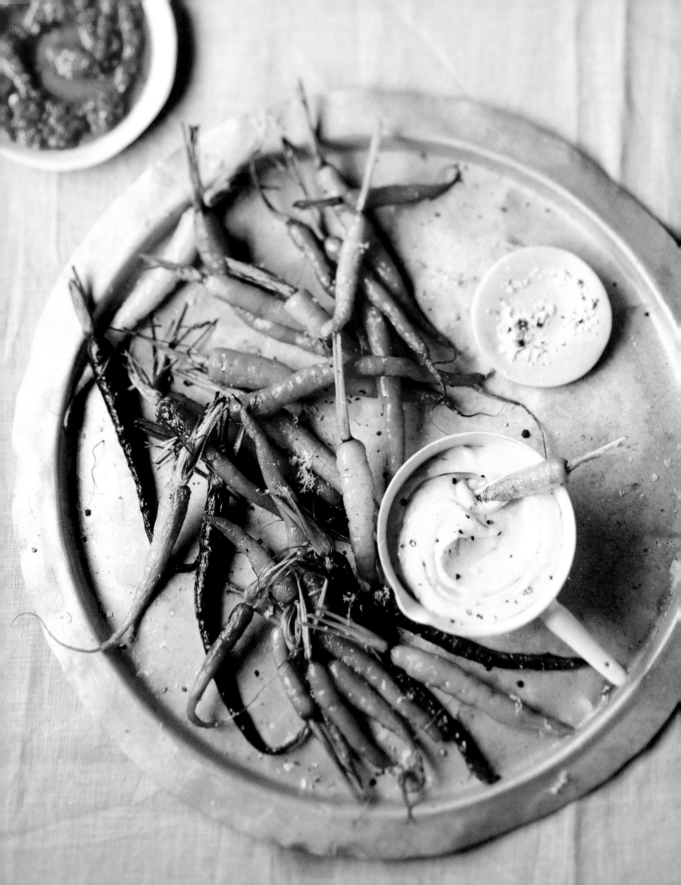

HUMMUS WITH HARISSA AND ROASTED CARROT DIPPERS

This is quite simply the most delicious hummus ever made (not that I'm confident or anything). The baking soda does something magical to the chickpeas to make a creamy, smooth finish every time. The homemade harissa gives it a fiery kick, which is perfect with the sweetness of the roasted carrot dippers. Although soaking dried chickpeas may seem like a laborious process, you will thank me when you try the end result.

serves 4
2 tablespoons Homemade Harissa
   (page 185)

for the hummus
1¼ cups dried chickpeas (garbanzo beans)
1 tsp baking soda
1 cup plus 2 tbsp tahini paste
4 garlic cloves, crushed
pinch of salt and ground black pepper
4 tbsp freshly squeezed lemon juice
1 cup ice-cold water

for the roasted carrot dippers
2 bunches of baby carrots, scrubbed clean
1–2 tbsp olive oil
salt

1. Begin by making the hummus. Put the chickpeas in a large bowl and cover with double the volume of cold water. Leave to soak overnight.

2. The next day, drain the chickpeas and transfer to a saucepan. Add the baking soda and cook over low heat for 3–4 minutes, stirring constantly.

3. Add 6 cups of cold water to the pan, bring to a boil and gently simmer the chickpeas, skimming off any foam or skins that float to the top. This can take 20–40 minutes. They are ready when you can press a chickpea between finger and thumb and it breaks gently. Check the firmness every 10 minutes.

4. Drain the chickpeas and blend in a food processor until you achieve a smooth paste. Then, with the food processor still running, add the tahini, crushed garlic, salt, pepper, and lemon juice. Slowly drizzle in the ice-cold water until you get a smooth, creamy paste. Transfer to a bowl and let it rest for at least 30 minutes before serving.

5. To make the carrot dippers, first preheat the oven to 350°F. On a baking sheet, drizzle the carrots with 1–2 tablespoons of olive oil and then toss. Sprinkle with salt. Roast for 20 minutes, until browned on the bottom and cooked through. Remove and set aside. Enjoy cool, with the harissa drizzled over them, and with the hummus for dipping.

GUACAMOLE

I love smashed avocado ... as does the rest of the world, these days. This is my fail-safe smashed avo recipe, which can be varied depending on what you are pairing it with. Try adding chili flakes, fresh sprigs of mint, or finely chopped bell pepper. The options are endless!

serves 4

2 avocados
1 garlic clove, peeled and crushed
1 large tomato, seeded and chopped
juice of half a lemon
half a red chile, seeded and finely chopped
small handful of cilantro, chopped
generous pinch of salt

1. Mash the avocados in a bowl and mix in the garlic, chopped tomato, lemon juice, chile, cilantro, and salt.

ROSEMARY PARSNIP FRIES

Parsnips are the perfect winter alternative to French fries, and the rosemary and garlic in this recipe add a flavorful punch.

serves 4

4 large parsnips
1 tbsp olive oil
¼ tsp salt
¼ tsp ground black pepper
1 garlic clove, crushed
3 rosemary stalks

1. Preheat the oven to 375°F.

2. Peel and cut the parsnips into long French fry–like pieces.

3. Scatter the parsnips on a roasting pan.

4. Pour over the olive oil, sprinkle on the salt, pepper, and garlic, and lay the rosemary sprigs on top.

5. Roast the parsnips in the preheated oven for 10 minutes, then carefully turn them over and return to the oven for a further 10–15 minutes.

MUHAMMARA (ROASTED RED PEPPER DIP)

I love traveling to Turkey partly because it's beautiful (our gym at the D-Hotel is one of the most stunning places that I've been lucky enough to visit) but also because I love Turkish cuisine. This dip was inspired by my travels there, and it makes crudités way more interesting.

serves 4

3 large red bell peppers

⅔ cup walnuts, toasted (plus a few extra, to serve)

3 tbsp olive oil (plus extra, to serve)

½ cup water

small handful of cilantro leaves, chopped (plus extra, to serve)

1 tbsp apple cider vinegar

half a garlic clove, peeled

1. Preheat the oven to 350°F and line a baking sheet with parchment paper.

2. Cut the peppers in half, remove the seeds, and place on the baking sheet. Roast in the preheated oven for 20 minutes, until slightly blackened. Let cool.

3. Once cool, slice the peppers and place in a food processor with all the other ingredients. Blend until smooth, adding water if the dip is too thick.

4. Serve with a sprinkle of walnuts and cilantro and a drizzle of oil. This is delicious with cucumber or carrot sticks, or spread over crackers.

HOMEMADE HARISSA

This harissa is a staple in my fridge. It's the perfect marinade for meat and is delicious in wraps. Once made you can keep it in a sealed jar for 2 weeks in the fridge.

makes 1 jar

10 fresh chiles

1½ tsp coriander seeds

½ tsp cumin seeds

½ tsp caraway seeds

4 fat garlic cloves, peeled and chopped

½ tsp sea salt

2 tsp tomato paste

2½ tsp lemon juice

1 tbsp olive oil

1. Blacken the chiles on a gas stovetop or lightly broil in the oven for 10 minutes. Remove from the heat and split lengthwise, discarding the stalks and scraping out the seeds.

2. Toast the coriander, cumin, and caraway seeds in a dry pan over low heat until fragrant, ensuring they don't burn. Transfer the toasted seeds, together with all other ingredients into a high-speed blender and blend until a thick paste forms.

WHOLE ROASTED CAULIFLOWER

Cauliflower is the new cult dinner-party dish. I'm definitely not complaining about that; it's such a wonderful vegetable and, when it's roasted, you can see why it's finding its way onto pretty much every trendy restaurant menu. This recipe is so easy to make and is a great addition to the Middle Eastern Bowl (pages 128–129). It also tastes delicious cold the next day, or chopped up and added to the Bodyism Frittata (page 136). In case you hadn't guessed yet, I love cauliflower.

serves 4
1 cauliflower (keep the stems and leaves on)
½ cup olive oil
Himalayan pink salt or kosher salt, to taste
3 tbsp toasted sesame seeds
1 tbsp chopped fresh parsley
1 tbsp chopped fresh mint
¼ cup pomegranate seeds

for the tahini dressing
½ cup tahini
juice of half a lemon
small handful of cilantro
¼ cup water
half a garlic clove, peeled
salt and ground black pepper, to season

1. Preheat the oven to 350°F.

2. Fill a large saucepan with water and bring to a boil. Place the cauliflower in the saucepan and leave to cook for 3 minutes.

3. Remove from the water and leave to steam dry for 10 minutes.

4. Place the cauliflower on a baking sheet, drizzle over the olive oil, and season well with the salt. Roast in the preheated oven for 30–40 minutes. Let it get really roasted and burnt in some places.

5. While the cauliflower is roasting, make the tahini dressing. Just place all the ingredients in a blender and blend it up.

6. Remove the cauliflower from the oven and place on a serving plate.

7. Drizzle with the dressing and sprinkle with the sesame seeds, parsley, mint, and pomegranate seeds.

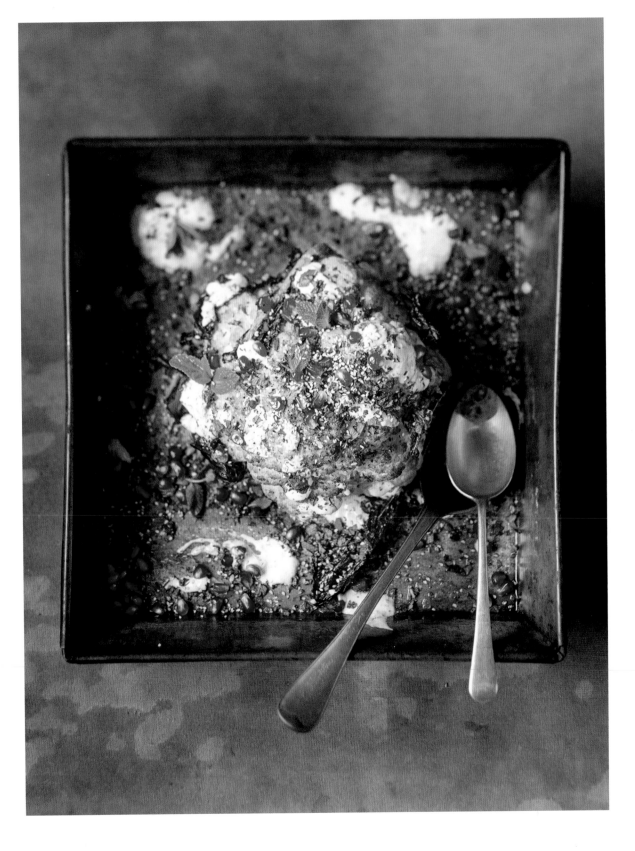

HEARTY ROASTED CARROTS AND AVOCADO

This dish is inspired by one of my favorite restaurants in New York City, ABC Kitchen. It looks really fresh and bright. Enjoy it with broiled fish or meat and some brown rice. Try to use multi-colored carrots, if you can find them, but regular long carrots look lovely, too. I would advise covering your roasting trays in foil before putting the carrots on, to save on sticky scrubbing later (you'll thank me).

serves 4

1 tsp cumin seeds, toasted and ground (or just ground, if that's all you have)
1 tsp coriander seeds, toasted and ground (or just ground, if that's all you have)
¼ tsp sumac
1 tsp salt
2 tsp fresh thyme
4 garlic cloves, minced
¼ tsp chili flakes
¼ tsp ground black pepper
1 tbsp red wine vinegar
4 tbsp olive oil
15 whole assorted carrots, scrubbed (there's no need to peel them)
¼ cup water
1 large avocado, cut into thin slices
2 tbsp toasted pumpkin seeds or sesame seeds
handful of any kind of sprout or arugula leaves
4 tbsp Greek yogurt (or more, to taste)

for the dressing

1 tbsp olive oil
1 tbsp freshly squeezed lemon juice
1 tbsp freshly squeezed orange juice
pinch of salt and ground black pepper

1. Preheat the oven to 400°F.

2. Make up your spice paste by grinding the cumin seeds, coriander seeds, sumac, salt, and thyme in a pestle and mortar or using a small food processor. If using pre-ground spices, skip this step.

3. Put the spices in a bowl and add in the garlic, chili flakes, pepper, vinegar, and olive oil; whisk together.

4. Spread the carrots out in a roasting pan (use two, if the carrots are too cramped). Cover them with the whisked spice mix and use your hands to make sure it's spread all over the carrots.

5. Add the water to the pan, just pouring it in around the sides of the carrots; this will help them cook. Cover the pan with foil wrapped tightly around it and put it into the preheated oven for 25 minutes.

6. Take the roasting pan out of the oven. The water will have evaporated. Remove the foil and put the pan back in the oven for about 30 minutes. The carrots should be brown and tender, but not falling apart.

7. Meanwhile, make the dressing. Combine the olive oil, lemon juice, and orange juice with the salt and pepper.

8. When the carrots are done, pour the dressing over them, then scatter the avocado, the seeds, and your sprouts or arugula on top. Finish with a few dollops of yogurt and dig in.

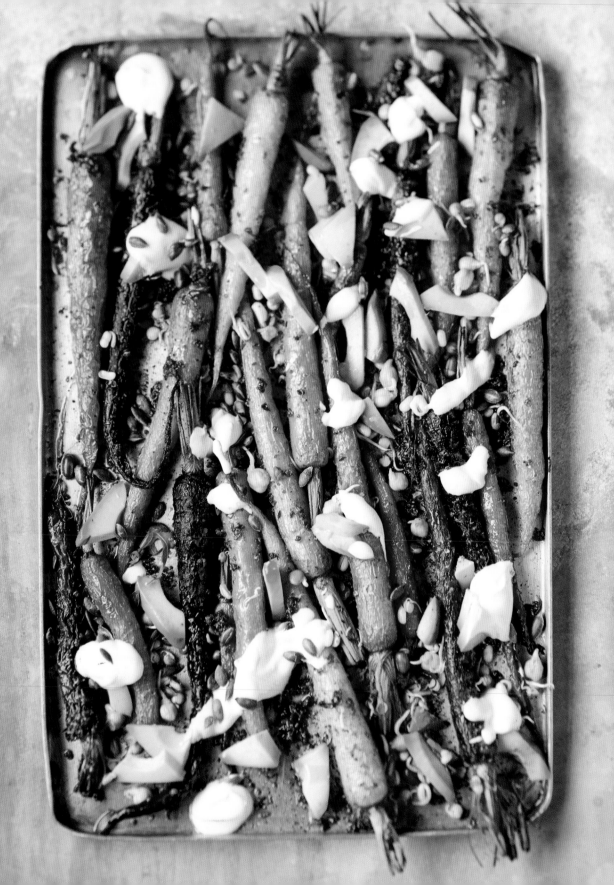

SUMAC FATTOUSH

This is the Lebanese version of a chopped salad. You want to scoop the seeds out of the tomato and cucumber, or else the salad will be too wet. Make the dressing first because the flavors will develop as it sits. This salad is wonderful paired with frankly anything, from fish and meat to vegetables. It holds up well in the fridge for a day or two.

serves 4

for the dressing

2 tsp sumac
1 tbsp warm water
1 small garlic clove, crushed
juice of half a lemon
1 tbsp extra virgin olive oil
½ tbsp white wine vinegar
pinch of salt and ground black pepper

for the salad

1 large ripe tomato, seeded and finely chopped
half a cucumber, peeled, seeded, and finely chopped
1 scallion, white and green parts, finely chopped
big handful of fresh parsley, leaves and stalks, finely chopped
handful of fresh mint, finely chopped
2 handfuls of baby gem lettuce, roughly chopped

1. Make the dressing first by mixing the sumac into the warm water and leaving it to sit while you prepare the rest of the components.

2. Add the rest of the dressing ingredients, including the sumac and water, into a jam jar or bowl. Shake or whisk to mix.

3. To prepare the salad, simply put the ingredients into a bowl and mix together.

4. Pour on the dressing about 5 minutes before serving, so the vegetables retain their freshness and the dressing soaks in. Dig in!

SWEET POTATO WEDGES AND CRISPY CHICKPEA BAKE

This vegetable dish is filling enough to be a meal on its own, or you can pair it with protein, such as steak or fish. The crispy baked chickpeas also make a great snack, too. Sweet potatoes are brimming with vitamins A and C and are pure comfort food.

serves 4

4 sweet potatoes
2 tbsp olive oil
1 tbsp honey
½ tsp salt
½ tsp ground black pepper
½ tsp crushed red pepper flakes
1 x 14-oz can chickpeas (garbanzo beans), drained, rinsed, and dried with a clean dish towel (the drier the chickpeas are before baking, the more they'll crisp up in the oven!)
¼ tsp smoked paprika
¼ tsp ground cumin
handful of cilantro, chopped

for the yogurt dressing

¼ tub organic Greek yogurt
1 scallion, chopped
2 tbsp freshly squeezed lime juice (or more, to taste)
salt and ground black pepper (optional)

1. Preheat the oven to 400°F.

2. Cover 2 baking sheets with foil—one for the chickpeas and one for the sweet potatoes.

3. Wash and pat dry the sweet potatoes—you don't need to peel them. Chop lengthwise into large, long wedges. Lay them on one of the foil-covered sheets and drizzle with a tablespoon of the olive oil and the honey, then sprinkle over ¼ teaspoon each of salt and pepper and all the red pepper flakes. Toss to coat, then arrange them in an even layer.

4. Put the baking sheet on the top shelf of the oven and cook for 40 minutes, or until cooked through.

5. Pour the chickpeas into the other foil-covered tray and drizzle over the remaining tablespoon of the olive oil, then sprinkle with the smoked paprika, cumin, and the remaining salt and pepper.

6. Mix everything together, spreading the chickpeas into an even layer, and put on the bottom shelf of the oven for about 30 minutes. After 12 minutes, give them a toss to ensure even cooking.

7. Meanwhile, make the yogurt dressing. Whisk the yogurt, scallion, and lime juice together. Add a sprinkle of salt and pepper, if desired.

8. Pour the chickpeas over the sweet potatoes. Add dollops of the yogurt on top and sprinkle with chopped cilantro for a fresh kick.

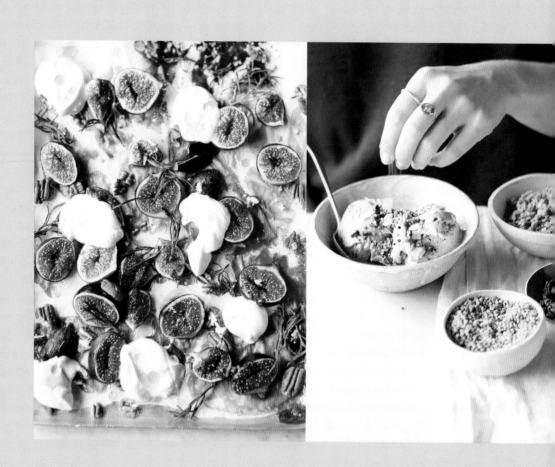

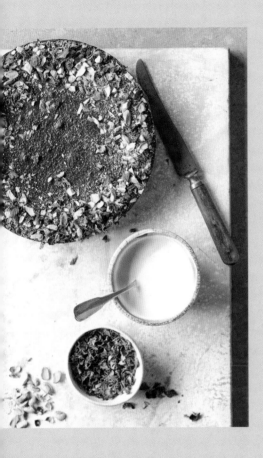

DESSERTS

Cherry Cobbler

My Apple and Mulberry Crumble

Coconut Carrot Cake

Persian Love Cake

Honey Cake

Molten Chocolate Pots

Bodyism Sundae

Broiled Figs with Greek Yogurt and Manuka Honey

Berry Coconut Popsicles

Spelt Crust Plum Pie

Comforting Coconut Rice Pudding

Super Seaweed Panna Cotta

CHERRY COBBLER

The cherries give this dessert such a lovely sweetness, which, mixed with the sponge, is pretty special. This is obviously an indulgent dessert, so please don't think you are being kind to yourself if you have it every day—but, when you do have it, enjoy it!

serves 8–10

½ cup butter, plus extra for greasing
½ cup brown rice flour
½ cup buckwheat flour
½ cup ground almonds, plus 1 tbsp for the cherries
½ cup coconut palm sugar, plus 1 tbsp for the top
zest of 1 lemon
1 tsp baking powder
1 cup almond milk
1½ cups pitted cherries, fresh or frozen

1. Preheat the oven to 350°F.

2. Grease an 8 x 12-inch baking dish. Melt the butter in a small saucepan.

3. Mix the flours, ground almonds, coconut palm sugar, lemon zest, and baking powder in a big mixing bowl. Stir in the melted butter and almond milk until thoroughly mixed.

4. Pour the mixture into the baking dish.

5. Place the cherries in a bowl and toss with the extra tablespoon of ground almonds. Scatter the cherry mixture evenly over the mix in the dish. Do not stir it!

6. Sprinkle with the remaining tablespoon of coconut palm sugar and bake for 40 minutes in the preheated oven, until it goes lovely and golden brown. A skewer should come out clean when poked into the center.

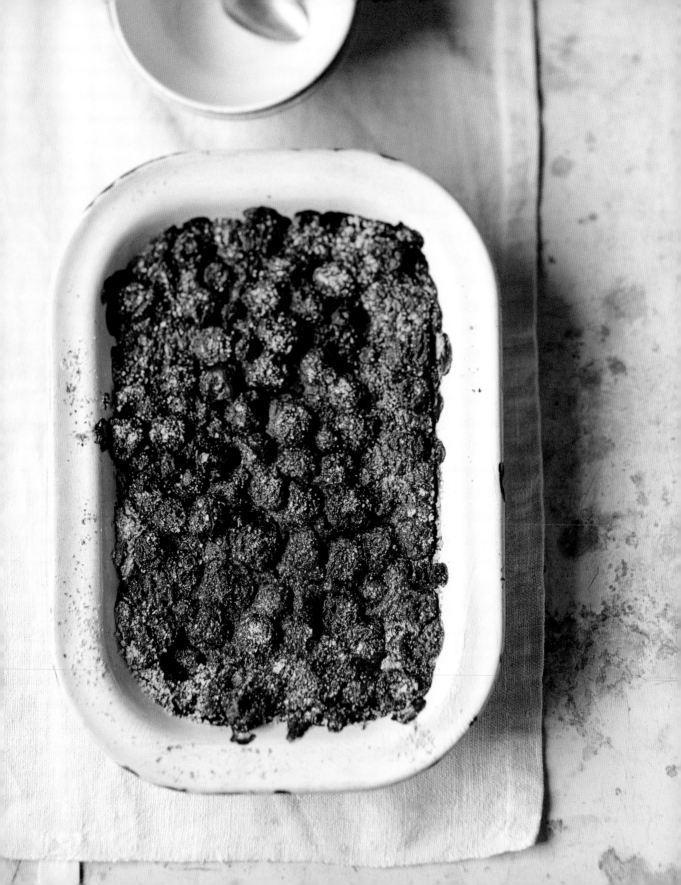

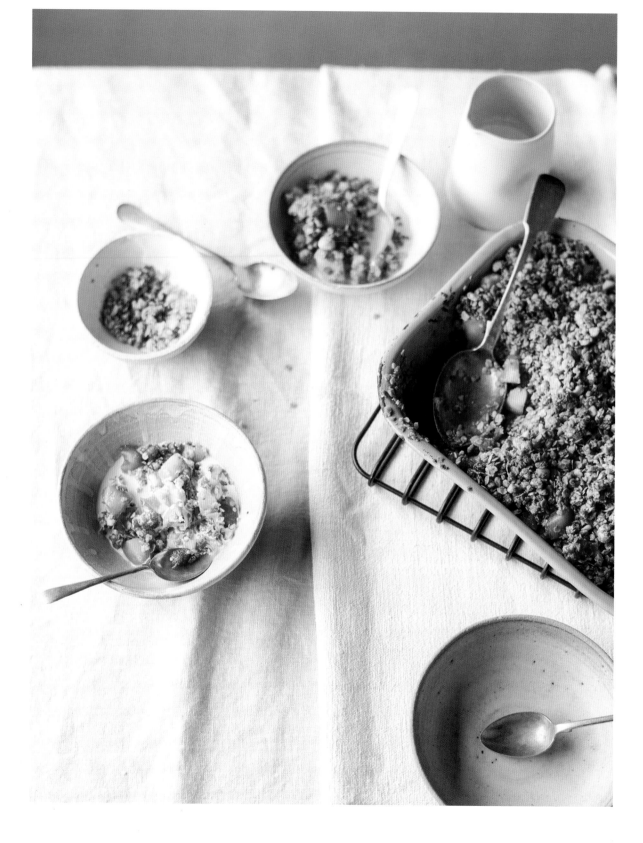

MY APPLE AND
MULBERRY CRUMBLE

When the apples are falling off the trees at the end of the summer, I make this with the kids. Sunday afternoons go up a gear when a crumble is cooking in the oven. As always, you are in charge, so if apples aren't your thing then swap them for pears, or lose a few apples and replace them with berries. Enjoy with a scoop of Bodyism ice-cream (see Bodyism Sundae on page 205).

serves 6

6 apples, cored and chopped (choose any variety; I like Braeburn best)
juice of 1 lemon
1 tbsp coconut palm sugar or honey
1 tsp vanilla extract
⅔ cup dried mulberries

for the topping

¼ cup hazelnuts, toasted
1 cup gluten-free oats
½ cup ground almonds
⅓ cup slivered almonds
½ tsp Himalayan pink salt
1 tbsp xylitol
½ tsp ground cinnamon
½ tsp vanilla extract
3 tbsp coconut oil, melted
2 tbsp maple syrup

1. Preheat the oven to 350˚F.

2. Place the apples in a large saucepan and heat over low heat. Add the lemon juice, coconut palm sugar or honey, vanilla extract, and mulberries. Let the mixture cook until softened—approximately 15 minutes.

3. Meanwhile, make the topping. In a food processor, blend the hazelnuts into a crumb consistency. Pour into a mixing bowl.

4. Add the oats, ground almonds, slivered almonds, salt, xylitol, and cinnamon and mix well.

5. In a separate bowl, mix the vanilla extract, coconut oil, and maple syrup and stir. Slowly add the wet mixture into the dry mixture and mix well.

6. Lay the crumble mix on a baking tray and use a spatula to pat it down so that it is densely packed.

7. Bake for 15 minutes in the preheated oven, until the crumble has started to turn slightly golden. Remove from the oven and let cool.

8. Pour the apple mixture into a baking dish. Using the spatula again, place the crumble mix on top of the apple mixture.

9. Bake for 15 minutes, but keep an eye on the oven. If the crumble browns too quickly, cover it with foil for the remaining cooking time.

COCONUT CARROT CAKE

This is the best free-from cake I have ever made—the coconut frosting is so delicious and creamy and goes perfectly with the lightness of the sponge. It's really important you use a good-quality, full-fat coconut milk. If you use one that is branded "light," then it's likely the added ingredients will mean it won't separate, which is essential for this recipe.

The coconut milk needs to be put in the fridge the night before and the bowl you whisk it in needs to be chilled beforehand, but, apart from that, this cake is really simple and easy to make for any occasion.

serves 10

for the sponge

3 tbsp coconut milk (use just the cream from the top of the can in the fridge)
¾ cup virgin coconut oil, melted
3 organic, free-range eggs, yolks and whites separated
1 tsp vanilla extract
½ cup coconut palm sugar
¾ cup dried shredded coconut
6⅓ oz carrots, grated
½ tsp salt
2 tsp ground cinnamon
1 tsp baking powder
½ tsp baking soda
1¼ cups self-rising gluten-free flour

for the frosting and topping

1 x 14-fl oz can full-fat coconut milk
1 tbsp rice malt syrup
½ tsp vanilla extract
1 tsp ground cinnamon, plus extra for sprinkling
handful of chopped walnuts

1. Put the coconut milk in the fridge the night before you make the cake, and put a mixing bowl in the fridge to chill, too.

2. Next, grease the sides of an 8-inch circular cake pan and line the base with parchment paper. Preheat the oven to 350°F.

3. Put the coconut milk, melted coconut oil, egg yolks, and vanilla extract into a mixing bowl (not the one in the fridge), and whisk together until combined.

4. Mix together the coconut palm sugar, dried shredded coconut, carrots, salt, cinnamon, baking powder, baking soda, and flour until well combined. Add the coconut milk mixture and whisk together until no lumps remain.

5. Whisk the egg whites in a separate bowl until they are stiff and remain in the bowl when it is held upside down.

6. Fold the egg whites into the cake mixture with a metal spoon. "Fold" is the key word, here. You want to get as much air into the cake as possible to make it light and fluffy.

7. Pour the mixture into the cake pan and place in the preheated oven. Bake for 35–40 minutes or until an inserted skewer comes out clean.

8. While the cake is in the oven, start making the coconut frosting. Place the thick cream from the can of coconut milk into the chilled mixing bowl. Add in the rice malt syrup and vanilla extract and whisk until the cream looks smooth and fluffy. Set aside in the fridge to firm up.

9. When the cake has finished in the oven, leave it to cool in the pan for 5 minutes, then turn it out onto a wire rack and let cool. Once fully cool, spread an even layer of frosting on the cake.

10. Dust with extra cinnamon and sprinkle the chopped walnuts on the top.

PERSIAN LOVE CAKE

This delicious spiced dessert is the perfect celebration cake, dinner-party dessert, or scrumptious treat. The Middle Eastern spices give it a rich, complex flavor, which, combined with the gooey texture, creates an indulgent, satisfying cake. Serve this with a spoon of Greek yogurt (ideally to someone you love or fancy) as a whole lot of love goes into this cake.

serves 6-8

2 cups ground almonds
1¼ cups coconut palm sugar
½ tsp Himalayan pink salt
⅓ cup unsalted butter, chilled
1 organic, free-range egg
½ cup organic Greek yogurt, plus extra
　to serve
½ tsp ground cinnamon
½ tsp ground nutmeg
½ tsp ground cardamom
2 tbsp shelled pistachios, roughly chopped
2 tbsp edible rose petals, to garnish (not
　essential, but beautiful)

1. Preheat the oven to 350°F.

2. Grease the sides of a 7-inch springform cake pan and line the base with parchment paper.

3. Mix the ground almonds, sugar, and salt in a bowl to combine evenly. Add the chilled butter and rub with your fingertips until the mixture resembles coarse breadcrumbs.

4. Spoon half the mixture into the prepared pan and press down firmly to cover the base evenly, as if you were making a cheesecake.

5. Add the egg, yogurt, and spices to the remaining mixture and beat with a wooden spoon until smooth and creamy. Pour this mixture over the prepared base and sprinkle the chopped pistachios around the edge of the cake.

6. Bake until golden brown and just set, approximately 30 minutes.

7. Let cool completely in the pan on a wire rack, before removing from the pan and transferring to a serving plate.

8. Sprinkle with rose petals (if using) and serve with an extra dollop of Greek yogurt on the side.

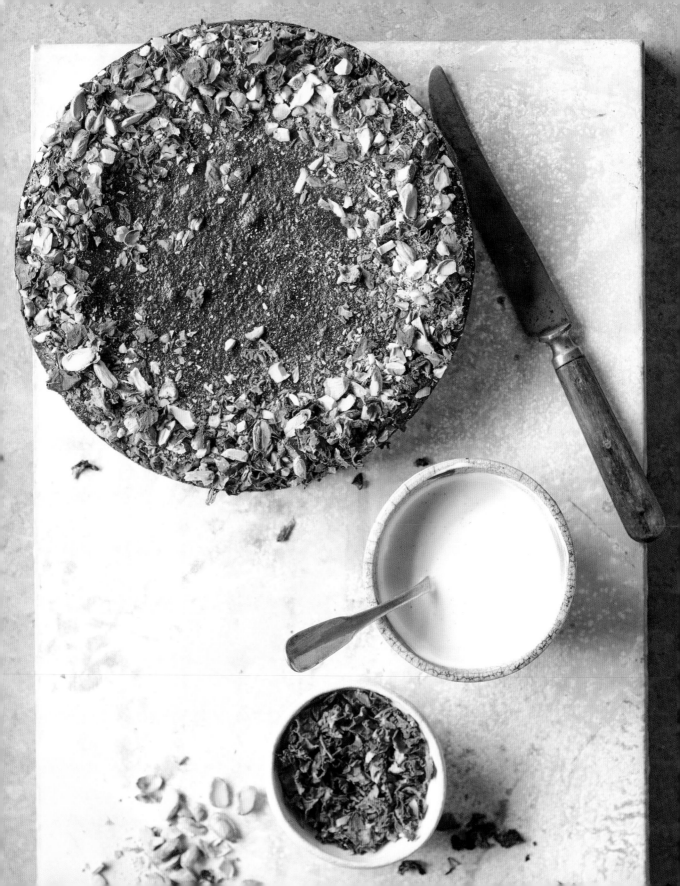

HONEY CAKE

This is one of Chrissy's favorites. The texture of the cake is so moist and we love it with a big pot of coffee. If blueberries aren't your thing, swap them for another berry or any fruit of your choice.

serves 8–10

4 tbsp good-quality olive oil, plus extra
   for greasing
2¼ cups ground almonds
1 tsp baking powder
½ tsp baking soda
½ tsp ground cinnamon
½ tsp ground ginger
½ tsp Himalayan pink salt
3 organic, free-range eggs, beaten
⅔ cup acacia honey, plus 1 tbsp for the glaze
1 lemon (zest and juice)
1¾ cups blueberries
½ cup toasted pistachios, chopped

1. Preheat the oven to 350°F. Using olive oil, grease the sides of a 9-inch springform cake pan and line the base with parchment paper.

2. Mix together the ground almonds, baking powder, baking soda, cinnamon, ginger, and salt.

3. Mix together the beaten eggs, honey, olive oil, and lemon zest. Add to the dry ingredients and mix well, until combined, then gently fold in the blueberries. Pour the mixture into the prepared cake pan.

4. Bake for 55–60 minutes in the preheated oven, until the cake is deeply golden brown and the center is firm to the touch (and a skewer inserted into the middle comes out clean). If the top of the cake browns too quickly, just cover it with foil and bake for the remaining time. Leave the cake in its pan and place on a wire rack to cool.

5. Slice the lemon in half and squeeze out the juice from both halves. Combine the lemon juice with the extra honey in a small saucepan and warm over low heat. Stir until well combined. Brush the glaze over the warm cake.

6. Once the cake is cool, remove it from the pan, sprinkle with the chopped pistachios, and serve.

MOLTEN CHOCOLATE POTS

I love a chocolate pudding. This molten pot is extremely indulgent and has all the satisfaction, without all the sugar. The outside edge holds it shape and, when you cut into the middle, the chocolate oozes out. For this recipe, you will need two large ramekins or three smaller ones.

serves 2–3
½ cup cacao powder, plus extra for dusting
2 tbsp arrowroot powder
1 tbsp xylitol
1 tsp vanilla bean powder
½ cup coconut oil, plus extra for greasing
2 tbsp cacao butter
½ cup maple syrup
2 organic, free-range eggs, plus 1 additional yolk
¼ tsp Himalayan pink salt

1. Preheat the oven to 350°F.

2. In a bowl, combine the cacao, arrowroot, xylitol, and vanilla powder, and set aside.

3. Put a small saucepan over low heat and melt the coconut oil, cacao butter, and maple syrup. Once melted and combined, pour into the dry ingredients and mix well.

4. Add the two whole eggs and additional yolk and whisk to incorporate.

5. Grease and line the ramekins with coconut oil and spoon in the mixture. Place in the fridge for 10–15 minutes.

6. Once chilled, bake for 10 minutes in the preheated oven. Remove and let stand for 1 minute.

7. Ease them out of the ramekins onto plates and dust with cacao powder.

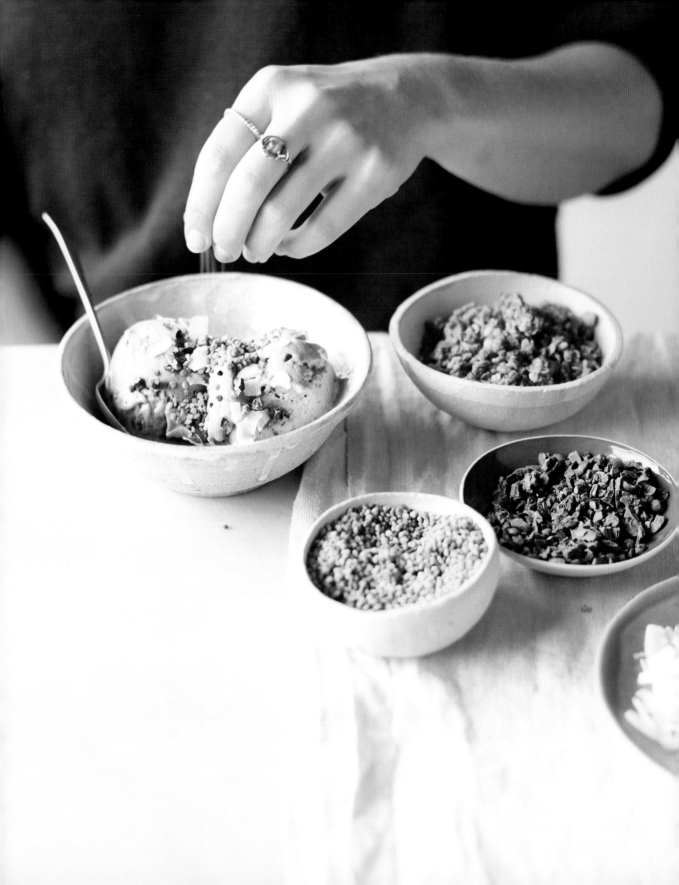

BODYISM SUNDAE

I've always had a thing for ice cream. As I've got older and more in tune with my body, I've realized that a mountain of ice-cream makes me hysterical—I can't handle all that sugar. So, when I discovered how easy it is to make ice-cream that is just as delicious, without all the unnecessary, toxic, refined sugar, I felt (and continue to feel) extremely smug. Now I'm sharing my secret. The trick here is to remember it's all about the toppings, so pile it high (and mindfully) with all the extras.

serves 4

4 bananas, peeled, sliced, and frozen
2 tbsp rice milk
1 scoop Bodyism Protein Excellence (or, if you want a stronger chocolate flavor, go for Body Brilliance)—if you don't have the supplements, then don't worry!
1 tbsp cacao
1 tsp ground cinnamon
2 tbsp almond butter
pinch of salt

for the toppings

Simply Granola (page 102)
cacao nibs
toasted coconut flakes
goji berries
mulberries
chunks of Bodyism Cookies, if you want extra indulgence (page 176)
The list could go on and on!

1. In a blender, mix the bananas and rice milk until you have a smooth consistency.

2. Add the Bodyism supplement, cacao, cinnamon, almond butter, and salt. Mix again.

3. Transfer to a freezer-proof container and freeze for 1 hour.

4. Scoop and serve, covered with all the toppings!

BROILED FIGS WITH GREEK YOGURT AND MANUKA HONEY

This is such a simple dessert, but whenever I make it, it reminds me that, if you choose delicious, good-quality ingredients, you don't need to do anything fancy with them. This is a light, refreshing yet wholesome treat. If you like fruit for breakfast, then you can definitely include this as a breakfast option (although I'd add some Bodyism Protein Excellence to the yogurt, so you get a good dose of protein to give you energy for the day).

serves 4
4 large figs
2 tsp ground cinnamon
1 tsp maple syrup (optional)
handful of rosemary sprigs
8 tbsp coconut yogurt
2 tbsp pecans, chopped and toasted

1. Preheat the oven to 350°F and line a baking sheet with parchment paper.

2. Slice the figs into halves and quarters. Place them on the prepared baking sheet.

3. Sprinkle 1 teaspoon of the cinnamon over the figs and drizzle with the maple syrup. Lastly, lay the rosemary sprigs over the figs, too.

4. Place in the preheated oven for approximately 40 minutes, until caramelized and soft. Leave to cool for 10 minutes.

5. Serve each fig with 2 tablespoons of the coconut yogurt and sprinkle with the pecans and the remaining teaspoon of cinnamon.

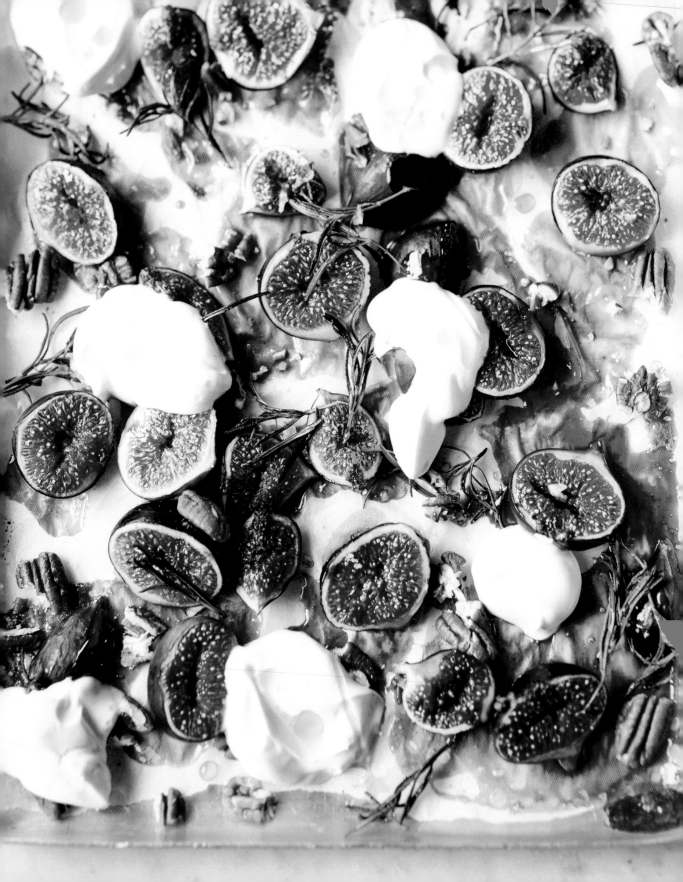

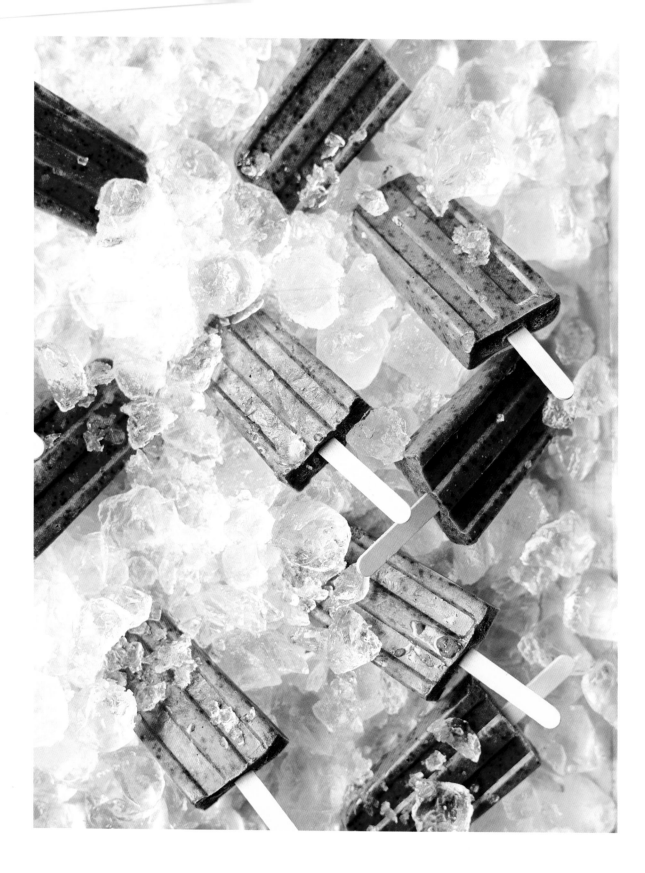

BERRY COCONUT POPSICLES

These are the kids' absolute favorite. Use this recipe as a guide and swap the fruit and milk as you wish! You will need standard popsicle molds for this recipe.

makes 12

1½ cups blueberries, frozen or fresh
1½ tbsp water
3 tbsp maple syrup
1 scoop Bodyism Berry Burn (page 219)
¾ cup canned coconut milk
½ cup almond milk

1. In a small saucepan, combine the blueberries, water, and maple syrup. Bring to a boil and cook over low heat until the mixture becomes quite thick. Remove from the heat.

2. In a small bowl, whisk together the Berry Burn, coconut milk, and almond milk.

3. Pour the milk mixture into the popsicle molds until they are half full. Spoon in the blueberry mixture to fill each mold.

4. Place in the freezer for 1 hour and then insert the wooden sticks into each popsicle.

5. Place the molds back in the freezer for another 5 hours (until they have become solid).

SPELT CRUST PLUM PIE

Victoria plums are beautifully sweet when they are in season, and there is nothing better than a delicious summer fruit pie served with a dollop of ice cream (see Bodyism Sundae on page 205).

serves 8

for the pastry

⅔ cup cold, organic butter, cubed, plus extra for greasing

2⅓ cups light spelt flour or all-purpose flour, plus extra for dusting

2 tbsp coconut palm sugar

pinch of salt

2 organic, free-range eggs

for the filling

2 lbs/5 cups ripe plums

4 tbsp maple syrup

2 tbsp cornstarch

1 tsp ground cinnamon

1. Grease an 8-inch pie dish with butter and dust with flour. Preheat the oven to 350°F.

2. To make the pastry, mix together the flour, half the coconut sugar, and salt in a bowl. Rub in the butter using your fingertips until it resembles fine breadcrumbs, then stir in one of the eggs and press the mixture together to make a ball of dough. Wrap the dough in plastic wrap and put it in the fridge for 30 minutes.

3. For the filling, cut the plums in half and take out the pits. Mix with the maple syrup, cornstarch, and cinnamon. Let sit for a couple of minutes so that the cornstarch can dissolve.

4. Remove the dough from the fridge and divide it into two pieces. Roll out one half on a floured surface until large enough to line the pie dish. Place the pastry in the dish, pressing it into the base and up the sides then trim the top to give a neat edge. Line the pastry shell with parchment paper, fill with baking beans, and blind bake in the oven for 10–15 minutes until starting to turn golden. Remove the parchment and beans from the shell and add the plum filling.

5. Whisk the remaining egg and brush it lightly over the sides of the pastry shell.

6. Roll out the remaining pastry and cut it into thin strips. Make a criss-cross pattern on top of the pie with the pastry strips, pressing the ends to the sides to seal. Brush the pastry top with egg, then sprinkle with the remaining coconut sugar.

7. Bake the pie in the preheated oven for about 45 minutes, until the pastry is golden and the filling is bubbling. Remove from the oven and let cool completely before serving.

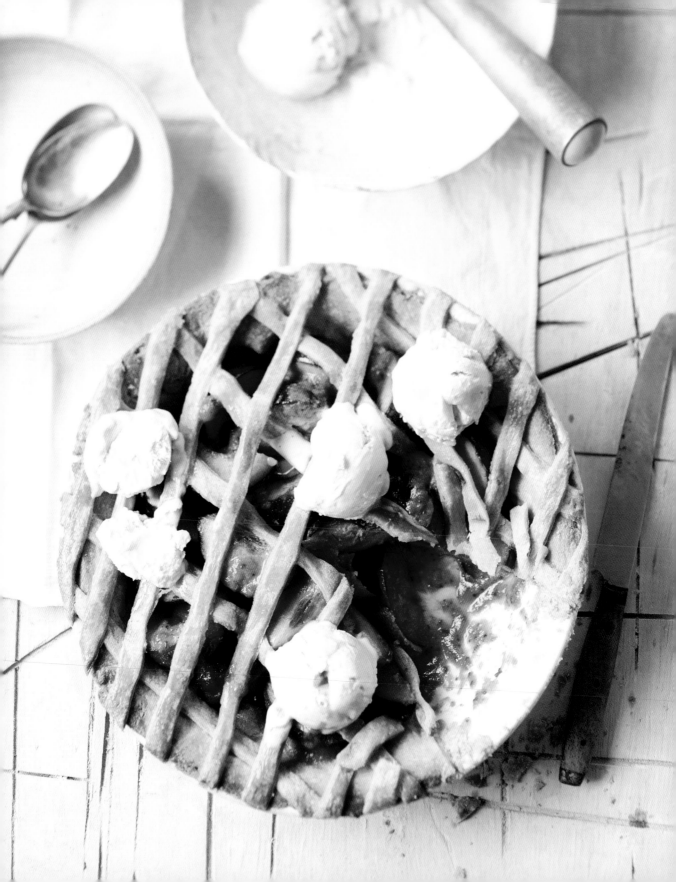

COMFORTING COCONUT RICE PUDDING

This is an old-school classic. My mother was way ahead of her time in her knowledge of healthy eating; she always tried to use whole, unprocessed ingredients, even when we didn't have a lot of money to spend. You can certainly make it with dairy alternatives, but if you fancy something lighter and dairy free, make it as instructed below. I love rice pudding with a dollop of fruit compote or some berries and slivered almonds—it's all down to personal preference.

serves 6

2 cups water
2 cups rice milk
1 x 14-fl oz can coconut milk
2 tbsp honey
1 whole vanilla bean
6 cardamom pods
3 tbsp dried shredded coconut
1½ cups short-grain brown rice
½ tbsp lemon zest
pinch of salt

1. Pour the water, rice milk, coconut milk, and honey into a heavy pan. Turn the heat to medium and allow the mix to come up slowly to a simmer.

2. In the meantime, split the vanilla bean lengthwise and scrape the seeds out with a sharp knife. Add the seeds and bean into the liquid.

3. Crush the cardamom pods in a pestle and mortar or with the back of a knife, and add them to the liquid as well. Bear in mind that you can take out the pods later, if desired.

4. Add in the dried shredded coconut, rice, lemon zest, and salt. Turn the heat down and allow this mixture to gently simmer for about 1 hour, stirring regularly so the rice doesn't clump together or burn.

5. Preheat the oven to 375°F. Once the liquid has reduced and the rice is basically cooked, pour the mixture into a shallow dish and put it in the oven for 15 minutes to firm up.

6. Take it out and cover the top of the dish with plastic wrap, ensuring the plastic touches the top of the pudding so that a skin cannot form.

7. Refrigerate until completely cool and set. Serve with compote, berries, ice cream or whatever you like!

SUPER SEAWEED PANNA COTTA

Irish seaweed, or carrageen moss, is world-renowned for its health properties and is a traditional remedy I grew up with for colds and flu. Normally made with dairy milk, this recipe is a vegan version. It takes minutes to make and keeps in the fridge for a few days, so it is the perfect make-ahead or last-minute healthy dessert. Serve with berries or fruit compote and a drizzle of honey.

serves 4
handful of dried carrageen moss
1 x 14-fl oz can coconut milk
1 vanilla bean, split lengthwise and seeds scraped out
1 tbsp honey

1. Run the handful of dried seaweed under cold water for a minute to rehydrate.

2. Put it into a pot with the coconut milk, vanilla seeds, and the split vanilla bean and gently heat to a low simmer. Don't boil it. Keep an eye on it and watch the liquid thicken for about 7 minutes, stirring it every so often with a wooden spoon.

3. Pour the liquid through a fine-mesh strainer into whatever bowl or little ramekins you plan to serve the panna cotta in. Add the honey and stir.

4. Let the liquid cool and put it into the fridge to set for 1–2 hours.

5. Once set, it is firm and has a panna-cotta-like consistency. It will wobble slightly when shaken.

6. Serve with whatever toppings you like; it's lovely with fruit compote and crunchy seeds.

BODYISM BASICS

THE ONLY RUB
YOU'LL EVER NEED

We all need a failsafe rub recipe for those nights when we're cooking something basic but are craving flavor. Make double or triple the quantity and store it in a jar, ready to whip out at the last minute.

---

serves 4
2 tbsp whole cumin seeds
2 tbsp whole coriander seeds
1 tbsp ground cinnamon
2 tsp ground ginger
1 tsp freshly ground black pepper
1 tsp ground turmeric

1. Toast all of the spices, both whole and ground together, in a dry pan for 2–3 minutes, until fragrant. If you only have pre-ground spices, then still follow this step.

2. Put everything together in a spice grinder or pestle and mortar and grind to a powder, unless you had only pre-ground spices to begin with.

3. Put the ground mix into a jar, where it will keep for up to 6 months. If using immediately, add a pinch of salt and cover whatever chicken or meat you're cooking, for aromatic flavor.

THE ONLY MARINADE YOU'LL EVER NEED

A delicious marinade is the way to give your meat, fish, or tempeh the x-factor. Learn this recipe so that you're safe if you're pushed for time but don't want to compromise on flavor.

serves 4

1 tbsp Dijon mustard
juice of half a lemon
½ tsp smoked paprika
¼ tsp salt
¼ tsp ground black pepper
3 tbsp olive oil

1. Mix the mustard, lemon juice, smoked paprika, salt, and pepper in a bowl. Slowly whisk in the olive oil so it emulsifies nicely into a creamy mix.

2. Pour this mix over chicken or potatoes before cooking, for a smoky, uplifting taste.

THE ONLY SALAD DRESSING YOU'LL EVER NEED

This basic salad dressing is my weeknight staple, perfect over any type of salad. For a twist, simply swap out the white wine vinegar for balsamic. Make a big batch and it will keep in the fridge for up to 5 days.

serves 4

2 tbsp extra virgin olive oil
2 tbsp water
1 tbsp apple cider vinegar
1 tsp lemon juice
1 tsp tahini
1 tsp tamari
½ Dijon mustard
pinch of salt and ground black pepper

1. Put all the ingredients into a bowl or clean jar and shake or whisk until the dressing forms a smooth, emulsified consistency.

2. Taste it and make the dressing your own by adding more lemon juice, a shallot, or a dash more vinegar.

3. Pour over salad greens, toss together, and serve.

Top Tip Add in some finely chopped shallot or garlic for a more pronounced flavor.

BEAUTY FOOD

Our Beauty Food skin-and-hair supplement is an all-natural daily elixir of super greens and marine collagen peptides, which can help prevent aging skin and will give you that much-needed glow. This is my take on the less impressive "green juice."

serves 1

1 scoop Bodyism Beauty Food
2-inch piece of cucumber, peeled
juice of half a lime
1½ cups coconut water
2 sprigs of fresh mint
3½ oz ice

1. Just blend it up in a blender and enjoy!

ULTIMATE CLEAN

This shake is a high-fiber probiotic formula, which contains slippery elm, wild rosella, and rice bran and is flavored with raw cacao, carob, and vanilla. The formula supports gut health by cleansing your insides and helps to keep you regular!

serves 1

1 scoop Bodyism
half an avocado
1½ cups brown rice milk
1 sprig of fresh mint
3½ oz ice

1. Just blend it up in a blender and enjoy!

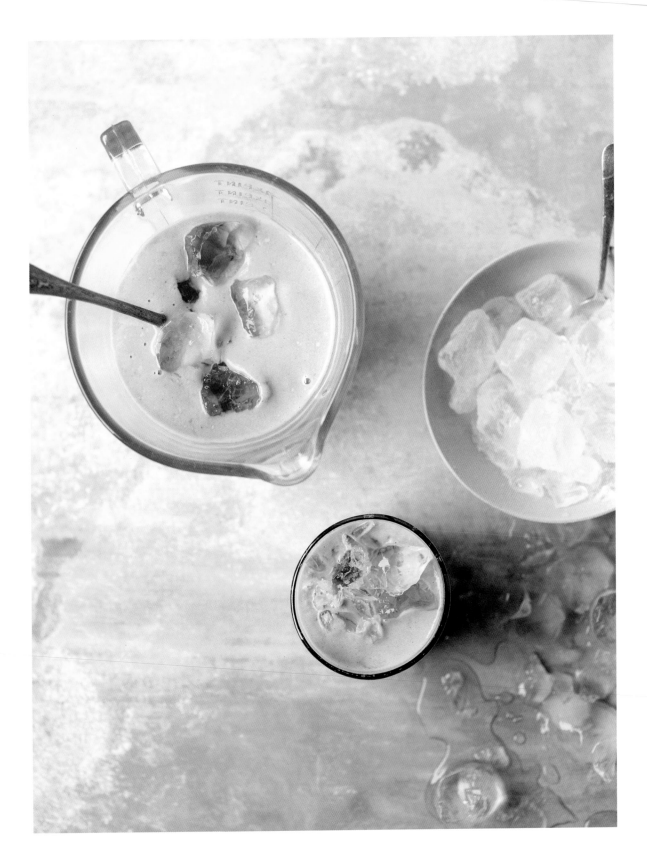

BODY BRILLIANCE

Our Body Brilliance supplement is an all-natural vegan protein supplement, which is packed with super greens, minerals, energizing herbs, fruit, and vegetables. We call it the "supermodel's secret weapon."

---

serves 1

1 scoop Bodyism Body Brilliance
1 tbsp almond butter
1½ cups almond milk
1 tbsp cacao
1 shot of espresso or 2 tbsp brewed coffee
3½ oz ice

1. Just blend it up in a blender and enjoy!

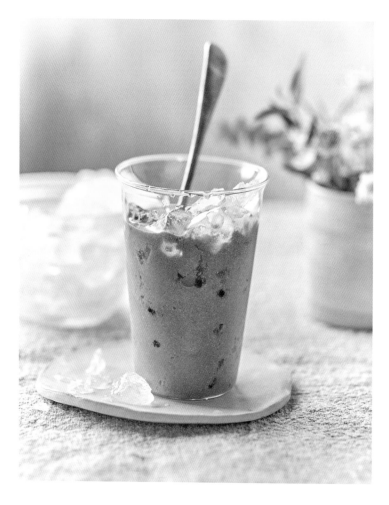

BERRY BURN

This is a deliciously thick post-workout shake, perfect for muscle recovery. Berry Burn is made with a range of different berries which are packed with antioxidants.

serves 1
½ cup coconut milk
1 cup coconut water
1 scoop Bodyism
1 cup frozen blueberries
1 tbsp chia seeds
1 tbsp smooth almond butter

1. Just blend it up in a blender and enjoy!

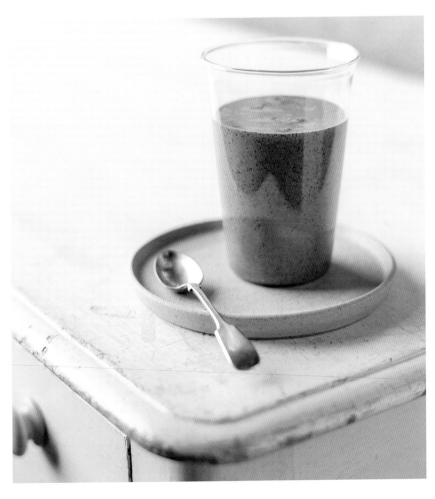

CHAI CASHEW MYLK

This is better than my childhood memories of warm milk and honey. The mix of spices reminds me of a cold winter's evening, which is why I love to make this for the kids and me to enjoy in front of a movie, with some Bodyism ice cream (see Bodyism Sundae on page 205). If you have the Bodyism Serenity supplement, try adding one scoop to the recipe.

serves 4

for the cashew mylk

1 cup cashews

4 cups filtered water

a couple of pinches of Himalayan pink salt

1 tsp raw honey

3 tsp ground cinnamon

2 tsp vanilla powder or extract

for the chai spice mix

½ tsp ground black pepper

2 tbsp ground cinnamon

2 tbsp ground ginger

1 tbsp ground cardamom

1 tbsp ground cloves

½ tbsp ground nutmeg

1. Soak the cashews overnight in a large sealed jar with half the water and a pinch of Himalayan pink salt.

2. In the morning, drain the liquid and wash the cashews in a strainer, until the water runs clear. Add to a blender with all the other Cashew Mylk ingredients and the remaining water. Blend for 3 minutes. Check the creaminess and add more water if it's too thick.

3. Now make the Chai Spice Mix. Combine all the spices together in a pestle and mortar and sift through a fine-mesh strainer. If you are using whole spices, make sure the ground mixture is very fine. Put in a sealed jar and enjoy for up to 1 week after making it. The Chai Spice Mix can also be used to make a delicious warming tea.

4. To make the Chai Cashew Mylk, add 1 tablespoon of Chai Spice Mix to the blender and blend again. Pour through a strainer into a bottle and keep for up to 4 days in the fridge.

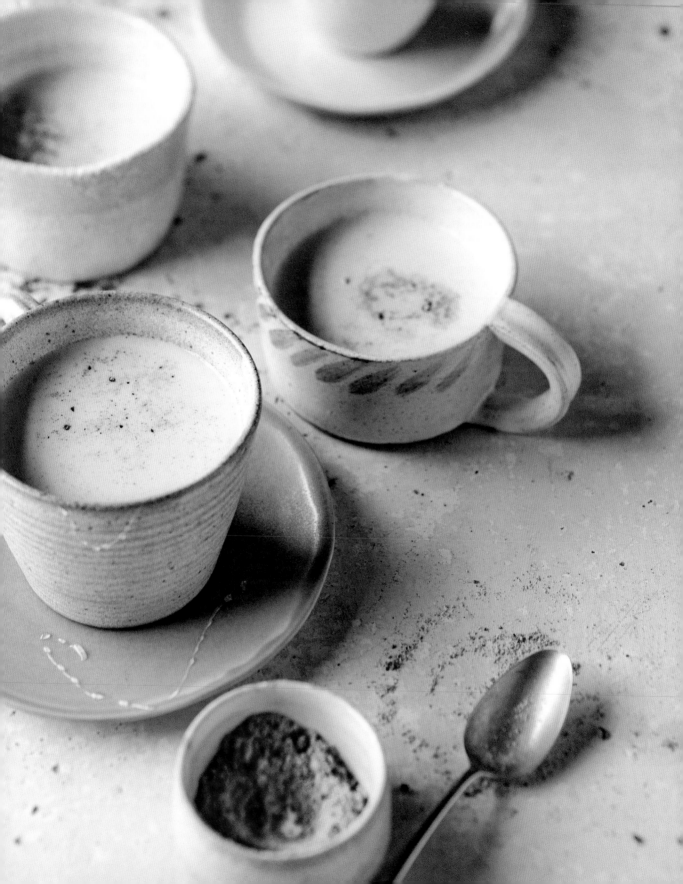

INDEX

açai bowl 96
addiction 20–1, 52–3
azuki bean mash 127
affirmations 16–17, 29, 83
alcohol 33–5, 81
alkalizing supergreen soup 137
almond and coconut pancakes 106
almond butter jam muffins 178
apple and mulberry crumble 197
avocados: avocado, tomato and chile salsa 112
   fish stick sandwich 130
   guacamole 184
   hearty roasted carrots and avocado 188

bacteria, gut 38
bananas: Bodyism banana muffins 181
   Bodyism sundae 205
Beauty Food 216
beet falafel 128
'being kind to yourself' 23
bell peppers: roasted red pepper dip 185
Berry Burn 219
Bircher muesli 101
blueberries: berry coconut popsicles 209
body, perfect 16, 41
Body Brilliance 218
bok choy and chile 124
bone broth 159
breakfast 31–2
broccoli: charred broccoli and chile 121
brunchy baked eggs 114
Brussels sprout salad, Asian 144
buckwheat: buckwheat, egg, carrot and mushroom crêpes 117
   the egg bowl 110
burger, the perfect 164
butternut squash: butternut squash hummus 129
   Moroccan tagine 152
   root vegetable mash 163

cakes 198–202
calories 38–9
carbohydrates 36
carrots: chai carrot chew-chew 105
   coconut carrot cake 198–9
   hearty roasted carrots and avocado 188

roasted carrot dippers 183
cashews: chai cashew mylk 220
cauliflower: cauli-rice 160
   cauliflower rice 126
   whole roasted cauliflower 186
chai carrot chew-chew 105
chai cashew mylk 220
cheat meals 41
cherry cobbler 194
chicken: chicken schnitzel 163
   harissa chicken 126
   leftover roast chicken pho 167
   perfect roast chicken 162
   poached coconut chicken 160
   sticky chicken thighs 148
chiles: homemade harissa 185
chocolate: chocolate cake 45
   chocolate soup 99
   molten chocolate pots 203
   pecan salted chocolate bark 174
circadian rhythm 79, 81
cocktails 35
coconut carrot cake 198–9
cod: ultimate fish pie 143
coffee 32, 80
cookies, Bodyism 176
cortisol 81
cravings 40, 44
curry, Keralan fish 161
cycling 51

dal, turmeric 147
dieting 30
digestion 38–9
dukkah-crusted salmon 144

eating out 33
edamame bean and ginger dip 125
eggs: Bodyism frittata 136
   brunchy baked eggs 114
   buckwheat, egg, carrot and mushroom crêpes 117
   the egg bowl 110
   Indian spiced eggs 107
eggplant: miso prawn and eggplant salad 132
energy foods 44, 45, 172
exercise 11, 21, 22, 45, 47–73
exhaustion 52, 87

falafel, beet 128
fattoush, sumac 190

figs, grilled 206
fish 32
   fish stick sandwich 130
   Keralan fish curry 161
   ultimate fish pie 143
frittata, Bodyism 136

garbanzo (chickpea): beet falafel 128
   butternut squash hummus 129
   chickpea dosa wrap 133
   hummus 183
   sweet potato wedges and crispy chickpea bake 191
gluten-free food 44, 45
granola 102
gratitude journals 82
guacamole 184
gut biome 38

habits, breaking 20–1
haddock: fish stick sandwich 130
happy bowl 126–7
harissa, homemade 185
hash, healthy breakfast 113
hazelnuts: not-ella 175
healthy eating 28, 41
honey cake 202
hummus 129, 183

immune bowl 120–1
immune system 79
Indian spiced eggs 107
injuries 52–3
Irish stew, slow-cooked 158
Israeli salad 128

kabbouleh 134
kale: kabbouleh 134
Keralan fish curry 161

lamb: zucchini lasagna 142
   lamb koftas 151
   Middle Eastern meatballs 156
   the perfect burger 164
   slow-cooked Irish stew 158
lasagna, zucchini 142
laxatives 38
legs, exercise and 57
lentils: turmeric dal 147
'listening to my body' 39–40

mantras 83

marinades 215
meatballs, Middle Eastern 156
meditation 80, 83–4, 85–7
Middle Eastern bowl 128–9
Middle Eastern meatballs 156
mindset 11, 13–23
miracle bone broth 159
miso prawn and eggplant salad 132
Moroccan tagine 152
movement *see* exercise
muesli, Bircher 101
muffins 178–81
muhammara 185

negative thoughts 17–19
noodles: leftover roast chicken pho 167
    Omega-3 bowl 124
not-ella 175
nutrition 10, 25–45

oatmeal, three-grain 100
oats: Bircher muesli 101
    Bodyism cookies 176
    granola 102
    three-grain oatmeal 100
Omega-3 bowl 124–5
organic produce 40–1
overeating 45
overtraining 52–3

pancakes 105, 106, 117
panna cotta, super seaweed 213
parsnip fries, rosemary 184
peaches, roasted spiced 106
pecan salted chocolate bark 174
perfect body 16, 41
Persian love cake 200
pistachio and raspberry medicine balls 172
plum pie, spelt crust 210
popsicle, berry coconut 209

positive thoughts 17–20
potatoes: healthy breakfast hash 113
protein 31, 43, 44
protein pancakes 105
the protein wrap 108

quinoa: kabbouleh 134
    Middle Eastern bowl 128

raspberries: pistachio and raspberry medicine balls 172
ratatouille dip 121
relaxation 52, 84
resistance bands 56
rest 52, 84
rice: comforting coconut rice pudding 212
    tuna poké bowl 154
root vegetable mash 163
routines, sleep 79, 81–2
rubs 214
running 51

salad dressing 215
salads 132, 144, 151, 190
salmon: dukkah-crusted 144
    miso-glazed 124
salsa 112
sexy stir-fry 157
shrimp: miso shrimp and eggplant salad 132
    shrimp summer rolls 168
sleep 11, 21, 31, 75–87
sleeping pills 87
smoothies 32, 44, 45
snacks, late-night 20–1, 81
soups 137, 138, 167
spinach: brunchy baked eggs 114
    wilted spinach, garlic and pine nuts 126
stir-fry, sexy 157
sugar 10, 31, 37, 44
sumac fattoush 190
sundae, Bodyism 205
supplements 41–4
sweet potatoes: sweet potato wedges and crispy chickpea bake 191
    turmeric, sweet potato, ginger and coconut soup 138

tagine, Moroccan 152
tartare sauce 130
three-grain oatmeal 100
tiredness 11
tomato and onion salad 151
trail mix 173
tuna poké bowl 154
turkey meatballs 120
turmeric dal 147
turmeric, sweet potato, ginger and coconut soup 138

two-week blueprint 88–91

Ultimate Clean 216

vacations 56

warming up 50, 60
weight gain 36, 38, 52–3
weight loss 56
weightlifting 58
worries 20
wraps 108, 133

yogurt 44

zucchini lasagna 142

Publisher's acknowledgements
Cover photography by Julie Adams and Kate Davis-Mcleod. Photography on pages 2–93 by Kate Davis-Mcleod and on pages 94–221 by David Munns.
Copy editing by Daniella Isaacs.
Recipe development by Julia Harvey, Daniella Isaacs, and Rachael McKeon.

FINAL THOUGHTS

Here's the bad news ...

Reading a book on how to change your life will not make a difference. Only you can make the difference. You can't plead ignorance anymore because the power is in your hands. You need to be kind to yourself.

Here's the good news ...

From this very moment on, you have everything you need to transform your life, your health, your body, your thoughts completely ... everything.

Remember, your past does not equal your future. Look at every past diet you've tried as a lesson which has made you stronger and more powerful. There is no such thing as failure—only feedback.

Knowing isn't enough—it's doing. You have an in-built, infallible guide within you, that loves you, that cares for you, and that knows you better than anyone else—that is you. You are your best expert.

Our bodies are incredible, magical, and wonderful. The problem is, we've been taught to mistrust ourselves, to numb ourselves through medication, toxic food, screen addiction, and any number of other distractions. This numbness brings us no joy, no happiness, and no comfort. We are uncomfortably numb. This book will introduce you to the most sophisticated, powerful, highly tuned technology ever created: you. Start with the two-week program, then learn to trust yourself.

Final three thoughts ...

1. Let go of shame and guilt.
2. Trust yourself.
3. Be unstoppable.

One more thing: make your world impeccable. If you say you're going to do something, do it.

Thank yous ...

As always there are so many beautiful people to thank. None of this would be possible without the incredible, selfless contribution of so many wonderful people.

To Chrissy and Nat, you're a constant source of strength and inspiration.

To my friend, partner, mentor, and big brother, Ferit, thank you for believing in me and thank you for making everything and anything possible. Thank you, Tevfik, for your unwavering support in everything we do. To Tom Koenig, for eating all the cheese toasties, and Luke and Chantelle, for always being there no matter what. Thank you, Adrian at Kruger Crowne, for making this all happen.

To our wonderful contributors; Rhaya, thank you for your intelligence, kindness, and genius—your passion and commitment is incredible. To Matt Bevan, for helping with the exercises and for being supremely dedicated. To Daniella, Rachael, and Julia, for the delicious recipes.

To everyone from the greatest team in the history of the universe, Bodyism, thank you for your dedication, positivity, and drive. To all of the people that have supported us over the past 10 years; our clients, our customers, our members, thank you so much.

To Emily Ezekiel, David Munns, Kitty Coles, and India Whiley-Morton, for making our delicious food look even more amazing. To Kate Davis-Macleod, our shoot at the D-Hotel was incredible and made us feel extremely lucky. Thanks also to Julie Adams.

And, thanks for my dad, for watching over me and making everything seem okay.

This is for my children.